KETO DIET **AND** INTERMITTENT FASTING

(2 BOOKS IN 1)

Perfect Combinations **to Burn Fat,**

Lose Weight, Cure Diseases and Stay Healthy

Amy D Morse

Published by Amy D Morse, 2020

Copyright

While every Precaution has been taken in the preparation of this book, the Publisher assumes no responsibility for errors or omissions, or damages resulting from the use of the information contained herein.

Keto Diet and Intermittent Fasting

LEGAL DISCLAIMER

The information in this eBook is not intended to replace medical advice.
No action or inaction should be taken based solely on the contents of this information.
Before beginning this or any other nutritional or exercise regimen, consult your physician to be sure it is appropriate for you.
The information and opinions expressed here are believed to be accurate, based on the best judgement of this author.
Readers who fail to consult with appropriate health authorities assume the risk of any injuries.

ALL RIGHTS RESERVED.

Table of Contents

Other Books from the Same Author

Best Detox Diets

Tired of Acne Skin?

30 Amazing Benefits of Turmeric

20 Detox Smoothie Recipes

To My Awesome Readers of <u>Keto Diet</u> and <u>Intermittent Fasting</u>

First and foremost I want to thank you for buying Keto Diet **and** Intermittent Fasting. I know you could have picked any number of books to read, but you picked this book and for that I am extremely grateful.

I'm sure it will add value and quality to your everyday life. Therefore it would be nice if you could share this book with your friends and family by posting to **<u>Facebook</u>** and **<u>Twitter</u>**.

I would as well like to hear from you, and hope you could take some time to post a sweet review on all the value you've gained while reading this Book.

Your feedback and support will help this Author to greatly improve her future Projects and make this book even better.

I want you, the reader, to know that your feedback in form of review is very important so if you'll like to leave a sweet Review, all you have to do is to scroll down to the bottom of the page and away you go. I wish you all the Best in your future success!

Thank You so much!!!!!!!!!!!!

Keto Diet and Intermittent Fasting

The greater part of your eating routine should be centered on Foods such as meat, fish, eggs, butter, nuts, healthy fats, avocados and vegetables that are low in carbohydrates.

What is Keto Diet?

Keto diet or Ketogenic diet: This is a low-carb diet with a higher percentage of fat intakes, in which the body produces ketones in the liver and utilized them as energy.

At first the fundamental general recognizable and available source of energy for our body is glucose. Whenever you consume any food that is high in carbohydrates, our body converts them into glucose, which increases the blood sugar and for its adjustment and the distribution of glucose in the cells of the body, the pancreas produces insulin.

Glucose can be defined as the simplest molecule in our body that is converted and utilized as energy, so it will be picked over some other source of energy.

Insulin is formed to process glucose in the blood by moving it all through the body.

Since glucose is utilized as an energy source, your fats are not required anymore and it will store up in the body. Commonly, in a normal, higher carbohydrate diet, the body will utilize glucose as the main source of energy. By decreasing carbohydrate intake, the body is resulted into a condition known as ketosis.

Ketosis is characterized as a condition of our body, which begins with a low level of glucose in the diet. With it, the body produces ketones, break up fatty acids, to provide us with a sufficient level of energy, nutrition for brain cells and organs.

The principal objective and ultimate goal of keto diets is to change us to the state of ketosis. It is important to know that it does not start with a low calorie intake, but rather with a low carbohydrate content in the diet.

Our bodies are exceptionally adaptive - as soon as they need glucose, it will easily switch to ketosis and begin to utilize fats as the main source of energy.

The best level of ketones and low blood sugar levels give us a great deal of advantages: from an overall improvement in health and a decrease in the percentage of subcutaneous fat, to an increase in mental concentration, energy level and vitality.

A keto-diet suggests a high fat content, moderate protein content and extremely low carbohydrate content.

The total nutrient intake ought to be about 70% fat, 25% protein and 5% carbohydrates

Advantages of Keto Diet

There are numerous advantages of keto diet ranging from losing weight and increasing energy levels to improving different medical health indicators. Beneath is the list of the primary advantages you can get from ketogenic diet.

1. Weight loss

The ketogenic diet changes your body to utilized fat as the major source of energy, so with a calorie deficit, your body is bound to squeeze and burn your fat layer. This is due to the steady level of sugar in the blood and, as a result of the absence of insulin emanations.

Studies show that at long run keto diet is much more viable for losing weight than any counterparts.

2. Sugar control

As discussed above, because of the practically complete absence of carbohydrates in the diet, you generally maintain an even level of sugar in the blood and try not to cause significant insulin outflows. This makes the keto diet an incredible solution for treating and preventing diabetes

3. Mental Core Interest

A high ingestion of fatty acids and the absence of sugar bounces in the blood is a great method to expand focus for a long period of time and to improve the focal point of attention.

Numerous Individuals notice significant improvements in mental activity at the end of fourteen to twenty-one days on a keto diet.

4. Increased energy and control food Cravings

Fats are very good source of energy that enables us feel fresh and energetic all through the day. Also, high-fat foods are extremely satisfying, and if you need to lose weight, it will be a lot easier to adhere to the required level of calories and control your food craving.

5. Lower cholesterol and Blood pressure

A ketogenic diet is a powerful approach of reducing weight and lower down "bad" cholesterol, which usually occurs on a keto diet, blood pressure is also normalized.

6. Insulin resistance

Insulin resistance is a violation of the metabolism of insulin in the blood. In specific, the pancreas starts to create more insulin for the distribution of glucose into cells than is required for a healthy person.

Increased in plasma levels of insulin can cause overweight and type 2diabetes.

A common explanation behind the occurrence of such a disease is a diet with a high content of carbohydrates which will result in constant jump in blood sugar levels.

7. Acne treatment

Individuals who have changed to a keto diet quite often notice improvements in their skin condition. Studies recommend that Acne is often occurred by glitches in glucose metabolism and its increased dietary consumption. Additionally, a reduction in the level of consumption of dairy products (particularly, lactose) in almost 100% of cases has a positive side effect on the condition of the epidermis.

.

Keto Flu and how to control it.

Keto flu isn't an infection that can infect only those who decide to go on ketogenic diet. This is the body's reaction to carbs restriction.

The most widely known symptoms of keto-flu are sugar cravings, dizziness, irritability, fog in the head and poor concentration, stomach pain, nausea, cramps, muscle cramps and sleep deprivation.

To control these, keep these simple principles

1. **Always Stay Hydrated Drink more water (with a pinch of unrefined salt).**

Hydration is essential, particularly when you are on a keto diet. If during a keto diet you don't drink enough water, you can easily dehydrate and experience symptoms.

2. Supplement your diet with potassium, magnesium and Sodium.

To get enough potassium, include avocados and leafy greens like spinach to your diet. Add a little of unrefined salt to every meal and to water to replenish sodium levels.

Magnesium is another essential mineral that can significantly ease your change to ketosis.

Even though you don't lose magnesium, while restricting carbohydrates, it is imperative to assist you prevent and completely eliminate cramps, improve your sleep quality and increase insulin sensitivity. Basically include almonds, pumpkin seeds, and spinach to your diet.

3. Consume more fat.

To enable your body to adapt, eat more fat. Fat gives Acetyl-Co liver cells, which they can use to make ketones.

4. Early in the morning, do exercise with low intensity.

As soon as you awake in the morning, fill the bottle with water and a pinch of salt, and go for a walk. The walk ought to be at a pace where you can effortlessly talk without gasping. It's desirable to walk about an hour.

As you keep strolling, you should feel much better and better and more and more awake. This is a type of low intensity workout that will help intensify fat burning, and you will not have to suffer from keto flu.

5. Reduce stress through meditation.

When you begin a ketogenic diet, you might be tenser and more irritable than usual. This is because of the way that your cortisol levels are slightly higher than usual.

To help lower cortisol levels and improve your overall well-being, it is ideal to do daily meditation

Consistently, for 15 minutes, simply sit quietly, breathing in and breathing out slowly and deeply.

The reason for meditation isn't to be thoughtless, but not to be distracted by the thought, but to focus on breathing. This is the way you train your mind that life is less stressful.

6. A sound sleep is the key to success.

Another approach to decrease stress levels is to ensure good sleep. Good rest is particularly important for keto diets. In the absence of this, cortisol levels will increase, which complicates keto-adaptation and Keto-flu. Always maintain sleep for at least 7-9 hours consistently every night, but if you feel tired in the middle of the day, meditate or lie down for 30 minutes.

To quickly fall asleep faster at night, switch off all lights (including your phone) at least 30 minutes before you proceed to bed. This will enable you transform your mind from work mode to sleep mode.

7 Easy Steps to reach Ketosis fast

Reaching the state of ketosis is quite simple and straight forward, but from start it might seem complicated and confusing. Here are what you have to do in order of importance:

1. Restrict your carbohydrates.

Majority of people in general tend to focus only on pure carbohydrates. If you really want great results, limit them. Always try to stay below 20 grams - 30grams of carbohydrates every day.

2. Limit the amount of protein intake.

An excessive amount of protein can lead to lower levels of ketosis. Ideally for weight reduction purposes take - between 0.6 g and 0.8 g protein per pound of lean body mass...

3. Worry less about fat.

When you are on keto diet, fat is the main source of energy - so always ensure you feed your body enough. Being on a keto diet, you don't lose weight because of cravings.

4. Stay Hydrated with water.

Attempt to drink around 1 gallon (3.8 liters) of water per day. It helps to regulate numerous vital body organs, and also control hunger levels.

5. Quit Nibbling.

Weight loss will in general improve when you have less insulin splashes during the day. Therefore constant nibbling can totally stop or slow down weight loss.

6. Start intermittent fasting.

Fasting can be an incredible tool for raising ketones all through the day.

7. Add Exercise.

To have great keto result you can add workout. If you want to benefit as much as possible on your ketogenic diet, consider adding 20-30 minutes of exercise per day.

Indeed, even a short walk can help manage weight loss and blood sugar levels.

Note: Always be watchful and ensure that you check the composition of the product you purchased on the labels. You will frequently discover hidden carbohydrates in foods that appear to be valuable on keto diet.

When you are on the keto diet, you can eat yummy, varied, satisfying, tasty and healthy foods

The 14-Day Meal Plan

Tips before starting

Make your purchases in advance and don't buy anything that you won't eat. Some items may deteriorate if you buy them ahead of time. In this situation, put them in the freezer or purchase a couple of days before you cook.

If you must take food with you to work, prepare it the day before for convenience. Check through the menu plan and always be ready to cook low-carb foods such as pesto, hardboiled eggs, crispy bacon, bone broth, mayonnaise and mustard e.t.c

If you don't like the ingredient that is presented in this menu, try as much as possible to replace it with another ingredient with the same amount of pure carbohydrates (pork for beef, blackberries for raspberries, etc.).

Always monitor your intake of sodium, magnesium and potassium to ensure optimum result.

Electrolytes are vital for your health and weight loss, most especially during the first few days of the keto diet.

This diet plan might not suit you; you are free to make some adjustments to suit your need. If you require less protein, reduce the amount of eggs and meat. Don't worry about a little excess of protein, it will not through you out of ketosis.

If you need to include more fat or less, focus on adding fatty foods and oils.

WEEK One Meal Plan and Shopping List

DAY 1

Total: 1650 Kcal

Carb: 14g Fat: 132 g Protein: 88 g

Breakfast:

Coffee with 2 tablespoons of whipped cream

Spinach frittata with feta cheese

Snack:

1/2 avocado with salt and pepper

Lunch:

4 leaves of lettuce

2 slices of fried bacon

1/2 cup simple egg salad (eggs, mayonnaise, a little mustard, salt and pepper to taste)

Snack:

24 raw almond nuts

Dinner:

2 cups chopped lettuce salad

2 tbsp. of Caesar salad dressing (without sugar)

170 grams of grilled chicken

3/4 cup casserole with cauliflower

Dessert:

90% of Dark chocolate 2 squares

NB: For a great taste you can include Lemon juice and Olive oil a Pink Himalayan salt, to each meal.

Total: 1636 Kcal

Protein: 88 g Carb: 18.5g Fat: 126 g

Breakfast:

Coffee with 2 tablespoons of whipped cream

Spinach frittata with feta cheese

Snack:

5 sticks of celery with 2 tbsp. spoons of almond

Lunch:

1 cup of sliced chicken meat

2 tbsp. of Caesar salad dressing (without sugar)

2 cups chopped lettuce salad

Snack:

1/2 half avocado with salt and pepper

Dinner:

1 piece of butter

2 tbsp. of grated Parmesan cheese or other hard

1 Italian sausage, cooked and sliced

1 cup boiled broccoli

Dessert:

90% of Dark chocolate 2 squares

DAY 3

Total: 1512 Kcal

Protein: 78 g Carb: 18g Fat: 119 g

Breakfast:

2 cheese fritters

Coffee with 2 tbsp. of whipped cream

2 pcs. fried bacon

Snack:

2 pieces of cheese

Lunch:

3/4 cauliflower casserole

1 Italian sausage, cooked and sliced

Snack:

1 cup of bone broth

Dinner:

2 cups raw spinach

1 tbsp. Ranch sauce (without sugar)

1.5 (one and a half) cups of pumpkin pasta with minced meat and spicy sauce)

Dessert:

90% of Dark chocolate 2 squares

DAY 4

Total: 1386 Kcal

Fat: 112 g Protein: 69 g Carb: 19.5g

Breakfast:

Coffee with 2 tbsp. of whipped cream

Spinach frittata with feta cheese

1/2 half avocado with salt and pepper

Lunch:

1.5 (one and a half) cups of pumpkin pasta with minced meat and spicy sauce

Snack:

1 cup of bone

Dinner:

2 cups raw spinach (14 calories, no fat, 1g carbohydrate, 2g protein)

1/2 cup anti-pasta salad

1 tbsp. Italian dressing (without sugar)

4 meatballs from dried tomatoes and feta cheese

Dessert:

2 squares of dark 90% chocolate

DAY 5

Total: 1649 Kcal

Carb: 18.5g Fat: 132 g Protein: 81 g

Breakfast:

2 pcs. fried bacon

Coffee with 2 tbsp. of whipped cream

2 cheese fritters

Snack:

1 cup of bone broth

Lunch:

4 meatballs from dried tomatoes and feta cheese

1/2 cup anti-pasta

Snack:

5 sticks of celery with 2 tbsp. almond

Dinner:

2 tbsp. sour cream

1 tbsp. chopped cilantro (optional)

1/4 cup crushed cheddar

1 Cuban pot (taco salad style)

2 cups chopped lettuce salad

Dessert:

2 squares of bitter 90% Chocolate

DAY 6

Total: 1604 Kcal

Fat: 122 g Protein: 89 g Carb: 19.5g

Breakfast:

Coffee with 2 tbsp. of whipped cream

3 eggs (scramble or fried eggs)

1 tsp oils

2 pcs. fried

Snack:

24 pieces of raw

Lunch:

2 tbsp. sour cream

1 tbsp. chopped cilantro (optional)

1/4 cup crushed cheddar cheese

1 Cuban frying pot (taco salad style)

2 cups chopped lettuce salad

Snack:

1 cup of bone broth

Dinner:

1.5 cups of pumpkin pasta with minced meat and spicy sauce

1 tbsp. ranch sauce (without sugar)

2 cups raw spinach

DAY 7

Total: 1609 Kcal (Fat: 128 g Protein: 90 g Carb: 18g)

Breakfast:

2 pcs. fried

Coffee with 2 tbsp. of whipped cream

2 cheese fritters

Snack:

2 slices of cheese

Lunch:

4 meatballs from dried tomatoes and feta cheese

1/2 cup anti-pasta salad

Snack:

1 cup of bone broth

Dinner:

2 tbsp. sour cream

1 tbsp. chopped cilantro (optional)

1/4 cup crushed cheddar cheese

1 Cuban pot (taco salad style)

2 cups chopped lettuce salad

Dessert:

2 squares Lindt 90% Chocolate

WEEK TWO Meal Plan and Shopping List

DAY 1

Total: 1752 Kcal (Fat: 144 g Protein: 89.2 g Carb: 18.3g)

Breakfast:

1 oz. Almond powder

4 oz. Coconut milk

1.5 oz. Blackberry, raspberry or strawberry; fresh or frozen

Snack:

1/2 avocado with salt and pepper

Lunch:

2 Boiled eggs

1 onion, lemon juice

6.3 oz Canned tuna

3.5 oz Crispy Salad

Salt and homemade mayonnaise, to taste

Snack:

24 raw almond nuts

Dinner:

3.5 oz. Avocado

1 tbsp. Olive oil

2 Large domestic eggs

2.8 oz. frozen spinach

Optional: crispy bacon pate, ham pate, or smoked salmon

Dessert:

2 squares of dark 90% chocolate

DAY 2

Total: 1615 Kcal (Fat: 129 g Protein: 89.2 g Carb: 11.2g)

Breakfast:

2.5 oz. Cabbage

Omelet with 4 oz. slow cooked meat

Snack:

5 sticks of celery with 2 tbsp. spoons of almond

Lunch:

2 Hard boiled eggs

1/2 Avocado

3.5 oz. Crispy salad, 1/2 onion

Snack:

1/2 half avocado with salt and pepper

Dinner:

4 oz asparagus, grilled

6 oz pork chops, grilled

2 tablespoons of grated Parmesan cheese or other hard

Dessert:

2 squares of dark 90% chocolate

DAY 3

Total: 1465 Kcal (Fat: 108 g Protein: 92.3 g Carb: 18.6g)

Breakfast:

5.5 oz. Stewed spinach

5.5 oz. Blackberry

1 Large egg

3.5 oz. homemade ham

Snack:

2 pieces of cheese

Lunch:

2.5 oz. Fresh spinach or other greens

7 oz. Shrimp, fried

1 oz. Green or black olives

Snack:

1 cup of bone broth

Dinner:

9 oz. Crispy tomato salad

5.5 oz. Slow cooked meat

Dessert:

2 squares of dark 90% Chocolate

DAY 4

Total: 1670 Kcal (Fat: 125 g Protein: 104 g Carb: 19.1g)

Breakfast:

1 oz. Bacon or ham

3 oz. Mushrooms

2.5 oz Cherry tomatoes

3 Scrambled eggs with a bunch of onions

3 oz. Stewed spinach, to enhance magnesium

Snack:

1/2 half avocado with salt and pepper

Lunch:

3 oz. Crisp greens, any one

5.5 oz. Slow cooked meat

Snack:

1 cup of bone

Dinner:

7 oz. Green beans, fried

7 oz. Large trout or salmon fillet, fried

Dessert:

2 squares of dark 90% chocolate

DAY 5

Total: 1544 Kcal (Fat: 127 g Protein: 69.4 g Carb: 17g)

Breakfast:

1/2 Avocado

2.5 oz. Cabbage

2 Scrambled eggs with a bunch of onions

2 oz. Bacon or ham

1 cup of bone broth

Lunch:

3.5 Crispy salad

2 Hard boiled eggs

1 Medium onion

Quick Avocado Salad:

1/2 Avocado

Snack:

5 sticks of celery with 2 tbsp. almond

Dinner:

9 oz. Crispy tomato salad

5.5 oz. Slow cooked meat

1/4 cup crushed cheddar

Dessert:

2 squares of bitter 90% Chocolate

DAY 6

Total: 1683 Kcal (Fat: 135 g Protein: 81.5 g Carb: 20.7g)

Breakfast:

1.5 oz. Blackberry, raspberry or strawberry; fresh or frozen

4 oz. Coconut milk

1 oz. Almond powder

Snack:

24 pieces of raw

Lunch:

5.5 oz. Cooked chicken thighs

3.5 oz. Crisp lettuce, onion

Quick chicken salad:

2 Hard boiled eggs

Snack:

1 cup of bone broth

Dinner:

6.5 oz. Steamed broccoli

3.5 oz. Baked salmon or trout, fillet

DAY 7

Total: 1788 Kcal (Fat: 149 g Protein: 74.8 g Carb: 17.5g)

Breakfast:

1/2 Avocado

5.5 oz. Stewed spinach

2.5 oz. Fresh berries

2 Large eggs (any preparation)

1 oz. Bacon or ham

2 slices of cheese

Lunch:

3.5 oz. Fresh spinach or other greens

7 oz. Avocado

Avocado, Bacon and Spinach Salad:

2 oz. homemade bacon

Snack:

1 cup of bone broth

Dinner:

6 oz Pork chops, grilled

2 tbsp. Grated Parmesan cheese or other hard

7 oz Asparagus, grilled

Dessert:

2 squares Lindt 90% Chocolate

Ketogenic diet drastically improve insulin sensitivity and leads to the loss of excess fat, which Permits you to effectively deal with type 2 diabetes and pre-diabetes.

Foods that you can eat on Keto Diet

- [ ] Bird
- [ ] Fish
- [ ] Seafood
- [ ] Offal
- [ ] Eggs
- [ ] Cheese
- [ ] Cottage cheese
- [ ] Butter Green lettuce leaves
- [ ] Celery stalks
- [ ] Onion
- [ ] Green beans
- [ ] Vegetable oils
- [ ] Broccoli
- [ ] Cauliflower
- [ ] Brussels sprouts
- [ ] Chinese cabbage(salad)

- ☐ White cabbage
- ☐ Zucchini
- ☐ Cucumbers
- ☐ Tomatoes (very few)
- ☐ Greenery
- ☐ Mushrooms
- ☐ Meat

Prohibited Foods on Keto Diet

All these foods are very high in carbohydrates or sugars.

So stay away from them completely.

- ☐ **Sweet dairy products**
- ☐ **Pasta**
- ☐ **Bran**
- ☐ **Potatoes, beets and other starchy vegetables**
- ☐ **Beer**
- ☐ **Products on fructose and sorbitol**
- ☐ **Milk**
- ☐ **Juices**
- ☐ **The nuts**
- ☐ **Fruits**
- ☐ **Powdered drinks**
- ☐ **Crab sticks and meat (imitation)**

☐ Soda

☐ Sugar

☐ Candy, chocolate, ice cream

☐ Desserts, pastries, cookies, waffles, etc.

☐ Preserves, jams

☐ Dried fruits

☐ Cereals

☐ Bread

☐ Starch

☐ Legumes

☐ Sunflower seeds

☐ Honey

Lists of the most Useful Nuts on Keto diet

1. Peanuts: It contains Folic acid and protein for the building of Nervous system and Cardio-vascular system.

2. Almond: It contains Potassium, Zinc, Calcium, Magnesium. It relieves headache and aid in digestion

3. Cashew: It contains Vitamins A, B1, B2, Fe, Ca and Potassium. It boosts immune system, Toothache and the Cardiovascular system.

4. Hazelnut: Contains folic acid, Protein, Vitamin E, Fe and B. It helps in brain activities, diabetes treatment and the cardiovascular system.

5. Pistachio: it contains folic Acid, Zinc and vitamin E. It removes cholesterol, Relives fatigue.

6. Walnut contains cellulose, Iron and Co. It helps in brain activity, and the cardio-viscular system.

7. Pine nut: It contains Vitamin B, C, E, M, and Zn It works for the treatment of seizures and against insomnia, fatigue, neurosis.

As you must have understood, that the most important food in the ketogenic diet is fat, this should make up 75% of the entire diet. These are, of course, the most useful fatty fish, vegetable oils (olive, coconut), nuts, cheeses and dairy products.

Proteins should represent 20% of the diet. You can get them from various types of meat, eggs and mushrooms.
It is of great important that meat products should not be processed such as sausage and sausages contain sugar. Alongside with proteins you have to remember fiber, because it is very important for a good metabolism.

On keto diet permit any green vegetables, as well as tomatoes. Carbohydrates should not be more than 5% of the diet, and they certainly must be "useful" and light.

These are, as a matter of importance, berries and organic products with low sugar content. Coincidentally about sugar: which includes any flour and, alas, pasta, you have to abandon them altogether. The same applies to any sweet beverages and alcoholic drinks.

Note: Regardless of the absence of calories restrictions, stay within your daily regimen. If you consume 4000 kcal daily, even the most effective diet will not bring results.

Before choosing Keto diet for yourself, make sure you Consult with your nutritionist:
keto ration and any other low-carb diets are dangerous for anyone suffering from metabolic disorders..

Meat

Since keto diet is a low-carb diet, meat is well tolerated in this nutritional system. Eat rabbit, beef, veal and even pork in small quantities: These foods contain a lot of protein and animal fats, which should be the basis of your diet.

Fish

Fish, similar to meat, fits perfectly into a carbohydrate-free diet. The "top choices" of keto diet are tuna, fat salmon, salmon and herring. This fish is extremely healthy, as it contains a lot of essential vitamins and minerals.

Chicken

We as a whole realize that dishes with lean chicken form the basis of any diet aimed at losing weight. So therefore, with keto diet: chicken is an essential product that contains a lot of protein and does not contain carbohydrates. Furthermore, it is always easy and pleasant to cook.

Zucchini

Zucchini is an exceptionally low-calorie (around 17 kcal per 100 g) product, therefore it is recommended to include it to the diet any forms of diet. It is rich in vitamins C and A, potassium and carotene. Low-carb diets are known to unavoidably lead to digestive problems, but zucchini assists speed up metabolism and normalize digestion.

Avocado

A low-carb, high-fat diet is incomprehensible without avocado. This product is supersaturated with healthful fats, vitamins and minerals, without which both a healthy diet and a diet would be inadequate.

Shrimp

These seafoods are highly rich in iodine and other beneficial minor elements, as well as vitamins A, D, E. Shrimps are incredible for a diet, and for keto nutrition- particularly on the ground that they contain important protein and beneficial Omega 3 acids.

Eggs

Eggs are the reasonable source of protein and healthy fats. Be sure to include them in your diet, examine the keto diet, since this product not just fits well into the low-carb concept of the diet, but also contains a lot of healthy microelements and vitamins.

A ketogenic diet can assist you with losing more weight than a low-fat diet. However, you will rarely experience hunger.

THE RECIPES

Keto Diet Smoothies

1. Morning Fruit Smoothie

Prep. time: 5 minutes / Cook time: 5 minutes / Serves1

10 Hazelnuts

1 Banana

1 tbsp. Flower honey

2 Kiwi

4 oz. raspberries frozen

Steps:

1. Combine all the fruits in a blender to a puree, pre-cut into cubes, except raspberries.

2. Beat the nuts in a blender (till small crumb remains).

3. Pour the smoothie into a glass, mix in honey, sprinkle with nuts, mix together.

PER SERVING

Calories: 656. Fat: 34 g. Protein: 13 g. Carbs: 77g

2. Invigorating Banana Smoothie

Prep. time: 5 minutes / Cook time: 5 minutes / Serves2

1 banana

6 prune

1 tsp. Cinnamon

17 fl. oz. Almond milk

2 tbsp. Almond oil

1.Put them in the blender, blend in with milk and almond oil, prunes, cinnamon and banana. Put them inside 2 bottles and put in a refrigerator.

2. If you are looking for a drink to enjoy, Perfectly stored them in the refrigerator for 2 days.

PER SERVING
Calories: 690. Fat: 45 g. Protein: 12 g. Carbs: 64g

3. Smoothie with Chia Seeds and Goji Berries

Prep. time: 5 minutes / Cook time: 5 minutes / Serves 4

2 tbsp. Honey
1 tbsp. Goji berry
1 tbsp. Chia seed

12 fl. oz. Milk

7 fl. oz. Yoghurt

2 cup Blueberry

1. Everything is very simple and straight forward.

2.   Put all ingredients in a bowl and grind until smooth.

3. Serve and garnished with fresh berries.

PER SERVING

Calories: 172. Fat: 9 g. Protein: 7 g. Carbs: 21g

4. Avocado Fruit Smoothie for Desire

Prep. time: 5 minutes / Cook time: 5 minutes / Serves1

4 oz. Fig

1 Avocado

1 Mango

4 oz. Apricot

1 Apple

4 oz. Strawberry

1. Aphrodisiacs are required here: make a blend of apricot,

apple, strawberry, fig, avocado and mango.

2. Put in a glass. Ready for consumption

PER SERVING

Calories: 473. Fat: 27 g. Protein: 6 g. Carbs: 49g

5. Spicy Tomato Smoothie with Pumpkin Seeds

Prep. time: 5 minutes / Cook time: 10 minutes / Serves4

2 Tomatoes

2 garlic, cloves

¼ tsp. Curry

¼ tsp. Turmeric

¼ tsp. Cumin

2 oz. Celery stalk

1 Beetroot

1 Carrots

2 oz. Peeled pumpkin seeds

1. Pure all in a blender, pre-cut the ingredients into cubes.

* As a replacement for tomatoes, you can make use of tomato juice.

PER SERVING

Calories: 117. Fat: 7 g. Protein: 5 g. Carbs: 10

6. Detox Effect Smoothie with Beetroot and Avocado

Prep. time: 5 minutes / Cook time: 5 minutes / Serves2

4 oz. Strawberry

1 Apple

Lemon juice to taste

½ Avocado

1 Beetroot

1 celery stalk

1. Pick small beetroot.

2. Wash all the Fruits

3. Cut into medium-sized pieces and put in the blender, beat.

PER SERVING

Calories: 487. Fat: 27 g. Protein: 8 g. Carbs: 57g

7. Chocolate and Nutty Smoothies

Prep. time: 5 minutes / Cook time: 5 minutes / Serves2

2 oz. Walnuts

1 banana

1 tbsp. Nutella

½ cup Milk

1. Cut the banana into pieces; add walnuts (6–8 pieces) add a cup of milk and a tablespoon of chocolate paste.

2. For 1–2 minutes, prepared to smooth with chocolate chips.

* Nutella can be substitute with half melted chocolate bar.

From nuts, you can use hazelnuts.

PER SERVING

Calories: 351. Fat: 23 g. Protein: 8 g. Carbs: 33g

Yummy Keto Breakfast

1. Keto Taco

Prep. time: 10 minutes / Cook time: 20 minutes / Serves3

Want to begin the day in an unusual way?

Morning keto is such an astonishing beginning to a delightful day.

Light and wonderful with a lot of bright colors and emotions.

2 tbsp. Butter

3 Bacon stripes

½ Avocado

8 oz. Mozzarella cheese,shredded;

6 Eggs, large

1 oz. Cheddar cheese, shredded

1. Preheat the oven to 375 °F. Put the foil paper on a baking sheet and spread the bacon on it. Cook it for about 15-20 minutes.

2. While bacon is cooked, put 3 oz. of mozzarella in a clean

dish and cook cheese over medium heat.

3. Allow for the cheese to roast around the edges (about 2-3 minutes).

4. Make use of a pair of tongs and a wooden spoon to make a cheese shell for tacos.

5. Repeat the same process with the rest of your cheese.

6. Cook the eggs in the oil. season with salt and pepper.

7. Place a third of the eggs, avocado and bacon in each hardened taco casing.

8. Sprinkle with cheddar cheese. Add hot sauce and cilantro if desired.

PER SERVING

Calories: 444. Fat: 36 g. Protein: 26 g. Carbs: 2.3

2. Keto Omelet with Goat Cheese and Spinach

Prep. time: 5 minutes / Cook time: 10 minutes / Serves1

2 cups Spinach

2 tbsp. Heavy cream

1 oz. Goat cheese

¼ Onion

2 tbsp. Butter

3 Large eggs

1 Medium green onion

Salt and pepper to taste

1. Try to cut the onion into long strips and fry it in oil until caramelized. Add the spinach to the pan and fry a little.

2. Remove the vegetables from the pan. Combine 3 large eggs, cream, salt and pepper together.

3. Pour the egg mixture into the pan and cook on medium heat.

4. When the edges of the omelet begin to fry, add a spoonful of spinach and onions to 1/2 omelet. Sprinkle with chopped goat cheese.

5. When the top of the omelet is ready, you can serve. If you like, garnish with onions on top.

PER SERVING

Calories: 621. Fat: 55 g. Protein: 37 g. Carbs: 4.8g

3. Chicken and Cheese Quesadilla

Prep. time: 10 minutes / Cook time: 15 minutes / Serves4

For lozenges:

Pink salt and pepper

1 tbsp. Olive oil for frying

6 Eggs

4 oz. Coconut flour

6 oz. Heavy cream

½ tsp. Xanthan gum

For the quesadilla:

8 oz. Chicken breast cooked and shredded

4 oz. Cheddar cheese, shredded

1 tbsp. Parsley, chopped (optional)

1. Mix in a bowl all the ingredients for the cakes, whisk well and let the dough relaxed for 8-10 minutes.

2. Heat the oil in a frying pan over medium heat and fry the tortillas for 2-3 minutes on each side or until well cooked. Set aside to cool down.

3. Heat a clean griddle over medium heat, put one tortilla, sprinkle with cheese, cover it with a lid and wait until the cheese begins to melt. Then add chopped chicken meat, extra cheese and cover with a second flat cake.

When the cheese has melted, remove the quesadilla from the pan, cut it into four slices and sprinkle with fresh parsley before Serving (optional).

NOTE: For the best results, use ground coconut flour. This will help with the texture, and you can make thinner cakes. Xanthan gum will also help make the tortilla strong and elastic.

You can swap fat cream with unsweetened almond milk. You can also reduce the number of eggs and add extra egg white. On the other hand, you will need to test and adjust the amount of flour used to obtain the desired consistency.

PER SERVING

Calories: 382. Fat: 31 g. Protein: 23 g. Carbs: 2.3g

4. Vegetarian Scramble

Prep. time: 5 minutes / Cook time: 15 minutes / Serves 5

This recipe is very easy to prepare with tasty avocados, tomatoes and cheeses will lift your spirits and energize you for great deeds.

1 lb. Tofu cheese

1½ tbsp. Food yeast

½ tsp. Garlic powder

½ tsp. Turmeric

3 Grape tomatoes

½ tsp. Salt

3 tbsp. Avocado oil

2 tbsp. Chopped onion

1 cup Spinach

3 oz. Vegan Cheddar Cheese

1. Wrap the tofu in several layers of cloth or paper towels, and gently press some water. Set aside.

2. In a skillet over medium heat, fry the chopped onion in 1/3 tbsp. Avocado butter until onion is soft and translucent.

3. Put the tofu in the pan and stir well with a fork.

4. Pour the remaining oil and sprinkle with dry seasoning.

5. Fry the tofu over medium heat, stirring occasionally until most of the fluid has evaporated.

6. Add the dice tomatoes, spinach and cheddar cheese and cook for a minute or until the spinach has faded and the cheese has melted.

7. Serve hot and store leftovers in the fridge for a maximum of three days.

PER SERVING

Calories: 211. Fat: 17.6 g. Protein: 10 g. Carbs: 4.7g

5. Burger with Guacamole and Egg

Prep. time: 5 minutes / Cook time: 10 minutes / Serves1

At times in the morning you may want a juicy burger with various spices. For that reason, I have prepared for you this fantastic recipe. Juicy meat, cheerful guacamole, an egg and 10 minutes is all you need to enjoy your favorite keto burgher. Everyone around will want the same.

1 Egg

1 tbsp. Olive oil (for frying)

½ tsp. Italian seasoning

5 oz. Ground beef

4 Bacon, slices

3 oz. Guacamole

Salt and pepper to taste

1. Get a small bowl, mix ground beef with Italian seasoning, salt and pepper. Make a small patty.

2. Put on the cutting board 4 strips of bacon crosswise, cutlet on top, and afterward wrap bacon around it.

3. Heat 1/2 tablespoons of olive oil in a skillet over medium heat, add the cutlet in bacon and fry 3 minutes (or more, depending on thickness) on each side.

4. Add the remaining 1/2 tablespoons of oil to the skillet and fry the egg, with the fluid yolk inside.

5. Put a guacamole, a fried egg on a cutlet, and, if needed, season with salt and pepper. Cut into half and serve immediately.

PER SERVING

Calories: 443. Fat: 33 g. Protein: 32.5 g. Carbs: 2.4g

6. Stuffed Avocado

Prep. time: 5 minutes / Cook time: 10 minutes / Serves1

1 tbsp. Butter, salted

1 Avocado, pitted and cut in half

3 slices of bacon cut into small pieces

3 Large eggs

Salt and black pepper, to taste

1. Place a large frying pan over low heat and add butter.

While the butter is melting, break the eggs into a bowl and whisk them, adding a pinch of salt and pepper.

2. Clean out most of the avocado pulp, leaving about 1.5 cm around.

3. Place bacon on one side of the pan and fry for a couple of minutes. On the other side pour the egg mixture and stir them regularly.

4. Eggs and bacon should be ready 5 minutes after adding eggs to the pan. If you find out that the eggs are cooked a little before the bacon, remove the scrambled eggs and place them in a bowl.

5. Mix the bacon and scrambled eggs together, and then fill the avocado halves with the mixture.

PER SERVING

Calories: 500. Fat: 40 g. Protein: 25 g. Carbs: 11g

7. Omelet with Mushrooms and Goat Cheese

Prep. time: 5 minutes / Cook time: 10 minutes / Serves1

2 oz. Crumbled goat cheese

2 tsp. Heavy cream

3 oz. Chopped mushrooms

3 Large eggs

1 tsp. Olive oil

Seasoning to taste

Garnish with green onions

1. Heat up olive oil in a pan. Fry the mushrooms until soft, for about 4 minutes.

2. As the mushrooms are cooking, whisk the eggs with heavy cream and a small amount of seasoning.

3. Pour the egg blend over the mushrooms and cook for about 2-3 minutes.

4. Add goat cheese. Fold the omelet in half and continue

cooking until the cheese starts to melt.

5. Serve it with spring onions or another side dish to your taste.

PER SERVING

Calories: 515. Fat: 39.5 g. Protein: 21 g. Carbs: 4.2g

Fat Bombs

1. Neapolitan Fatty Bombs

Prep. time: 10 minutes / Cook time: 15 minutes / Serves24

2 tbsp. Erythritol

½ cup Coconut oil

25 drops Liquid stevia

2 tbsp. Cocoa powder

½ cup Butter

½ cup Sour cream

½ cup Cream cheese

1 tsp. Vanilla extract

2 medium strawberries

1. Utilize a blender, mix all the ingredients (except cocoa powder, vanilla and strawberry) in a bowl.

2. Share the mixture into 3 bowls. Add cocoa powder to one, vanilla to another, and strawberries to third.

3. Pour the chocolate mixture into the mold and place in the freezer for 30 minutes.

Repeat the process with vanilla and strawberry layers.

4. Allow all of it to freeze for at least 1 hour.

PER SERVING

Calories: 102. Fat: 11 g. Protein: 1 g. Carbs: 0.5g

2. Chocolate-Coconut Fat Bombs with Almonds

Prep. time: 5 minutes / Cook time: 15 minutes / Serves12

3 tbsp. Coconut oil (melted)

24 Almond, pieces

1 cup Coconut chips

4 oz. Chocolate chips, no sugar

3 tbsp. Fat coconut milk

½ tsp. Vanilla extract

A pinch of salt

2 oz. Keto-friendly sweetener

1. Put 2 tablespoons of melted coconut oil, coconut milk, coconut chips, sweetener, vanilla extract and salt in a small bowl.

2. Share the mixture into 12 servings and place them on a baking sheet with parchment paper.

Put in the freezer for 5 minutes, then put on each fat bomb 1-2 things almonds.

3. Melt the chocolate chips together with 2 teaspoons of coconut oil in the microwave.

4. Remove the bombs from the freezer, pour each of the chocolate mixture and cool.

PER SERVING

Calories: 92. Fat: 9 g. Protein: 2 g. Carbs: 1.5g

3. Fiery Fat Bombs

Prep. time: 5 minutes / Cook time: 15 minutes / Serves12

1 tbsp. Black sesame seeds

½ tsp. Cinnamon

Pinch Chinese 5 Spice Blend

6 MCT powder, scoops

10 Liquid stevia, drops

1 tsp. Turmeric A pinch of black pepper

2½ fl. oz. Warm water

1. Combine all the dry ingredients in a small bowl.

2. Gradually add warm water and mix until smooth.

3. Spread the all the mixture evenly over 12 silicone molds, about 1tbsp. l on each.

4. Keep in the fridge so that the fat bombs are well frozen. Always store them frozen, otherwise they will quickly melt.

PER SERVING

Calories: 81. Fat: 8 g. Protein: 1 g. Carbs: 1.5

4. Espresso Fat Bombs

Prep. time: 5 minutes / Cook time: 30 minutes / Serves12

2 oz. Ghee butter (melted)

2 oz. Heavy cream

1 tsp. Vanilla extract

1 tbsp. Milk to your taste

Double espresso

4oz. Butter

2oz. Keto-friendly sweetener of your choice

A pinch of salt

1. Combine all the ingredients into a small food processor and whip at high speed until it looks airy.

2. Add sweetener to taste.

3. Pour it into molds and refrigerate for 30 minutes (or more if you wish)

PER SERVING

Calories: 61. Fat: 5 g. Protein: 1 g. Carbs: 1g

1. Almond Coconut Fat Bombs

Prep. time: 5 minutes / Cook time: 20 minutes / Serves10

2 fl. oz Coconut oil

2 fl. oz. Almond oil

2 tbsp. Cocoa powder

2 fl. oz Erythritol, to your taste

1. Blend almond and coconut oil in a microwave dish.

2. Warm the mixture in the microwave for 30-45 seconds and

mix until a homogeneous mass. Add cocoa powder and erythritol powder, and mix to complete the mix.

3. Share the mass into mini cupcake molds and refrigerate in the refrigerator.

PER SERVING

Calories: 89. Fat: 9.3 g. Protein: 1.5 g. Carbs: 1g

2. Pumpkin Fat Spice Bombs

Prep. time: 5 minutes / Cook time: 10 minutes / Serves9

3 fl. oz. Pumpkin puree

2 tbsp. MCT oils

2 tsp. Cinnamon, ground

8 oz. Raw cashews

4 oz. Raw macadamia nuts

4 oz. Coconut chips

2 tsp. Ginger, ground

Neutral oil (avocado oil)

1.Combine all the ingredients in a food processor and mix to form a dough.

2. Grease your Palms with neutral oil, such as avocado oil. Make use of spoon, take about 3.5 -4 oz. of the batter into lightly oiled hands and form a ball. Postpone and repeat the process (about 9 "bombs" in total).

3. Garnish fat bombs with savory coconut chips.

4. Such fatty bombs can be eaten immediately, or stored in a refrigerator / freezer.

PER SERVING

Calories: 217. Fat: 19 g. Protein: 5 g. Carbs: 5g

3. Cheese Fat Bombs in Bacon

Prep. time: 5 minutes / Cook time: 20 minutes / Serves20

4 tbsp. Butter, melted

20 Bacon, slices

3 tbsp. Psyllium powder

1 Egg

8 oz. Mozzarella cheese

4 tbsp. Almond flour

Salt, to taste

1 tsp. Black pepper

1/8 tsp. Garlic powder

1/8 tsp. Onion powder

1. Microwave half of the cheese for 45-60 seconds or until it
melts and becomes sticky.
2. Heat the butter in the microwave for 15-20 seconds until completely melted, then mix it with cheese and egg.
3. Add psyllium husks, almond flour and spices. Mix again and lay out the dough in rectangle.
4. Fill the rectangle with the rest of the cheese and fold it in half (horizontally), then in half (vertically).
5. Trim the edges and form into a rectangle. Cut 20 square pieces.

6. Wrap each piece of dough with a piece of bacon, use toothpicks to fasten it.

7. Put each piece in bubbling oil and cook for 1-3 minutes.

PER SERVING

Calories: 93. Fat: 8 g. Protein: 5 g. Carbs: 1g

SALADS

1. Vegetable Salad with Bacon and Cheese

Prep. time: 5 minutes / Cook time: 10 minutes / Serves6

3 tbsp. Sour cream

2 ½ tbsp. Mayonnaise

2 oz. Blue cheese

4 oz. Lettuce

3 oz. Spinach

2 oz. Curly cabbage

6 slices of cooked bacon

12 pcs. grape tomato

1 Avocado, peeled and sliced

1.Get a small bowl, mix the sour cream and mayonnaise.

2. Mix with half the blue cheese and set aside.

3. Get big salad bowl, mix the remaining ingredients.

4. Spread the salad into portions and place the blue cheese dressing on top.

PER SERVING

Calories: 183. Fat: 16 g. Protein: 6.5 g. Carbs: 2.5g

2. Salad with Chicken Breast and Greens

Prep. time: 10 minutes / Cook time: 30 minutes / Serves2

2 tbsp. Pesto sauce

2 fl. oz. Balsamic vinegar

1 tsp. Olive oil

6 oz. Chicken breast

4 cup Spring greens

1 oz. Fresh mozzarella

¼ Avocado, diced

6 Cherry tomatoes

1 tbsp. Fresh basil for decoration

1. Prepare the marinade by mixing pesto, balsamic vinegar and olive oil.

2. Set aside a portion of the marinade for the salad, and pour the remaining chicken breast. Refrigerate marinate for at least 20 minutes.

3. Take the salad. Start with greens, then layered with fresh mozzarella, avocado and tomatoes.

4. Once the chicken is pickled, heat the medium-sized griddle and then add a little olive oil.

5. Fry each side of the breast for 7-10 minutes.

6. Slice the chicken breast and place on the previously prepared salad.

7. Pour the remaining balsamic pesto and add some chopped fresh basil.

PER SERVING

Calories: 306. Fat: 16 g. Protein: 25 g. Carbs: 6.5g

3. Salmon Salad

Prep. time: 5 minutes / Cook time: 10 minutes / Serves2

2 Sheets of lettuce

6 leaves, Fresh basil, finely chopped

½ tsp. Garlic powder

1 tsp. Lemon juice

4 tbsp. Mayonnaise

5 oz. Salmon

1 oz. Red onion, chopped

½ Avocado, diced

2 tbsp. Parmesan cheese, diced

1. Rinse well and clean the lettuce leaves - they will serve as plates.

2. Mix lemon juice, chopped basil and garlic powder.

3. Add mayonnaise and mix well. Set aside.

4. Fill each "plate" of lettuce with half of the finely chopped salmon, and then avocado and onion rings.

5. Top with evenly arrange the mayonnaise (earlier about 2tablespoons per serving), then place the parmesan cubes.

PER SERVING

Calories: 373. Fat: 31 g. Protein: 19.6 g. Carbs: 2.5g

4. Simple Cabbage and Egg Keto Salad

Prep. time: 10 minutes / Cook time: 10 minutes / Serves 6

1 lb. Cauliflower flowers

4 oz. Keto mayonnaise

1 tsp. Yellow mustard

1½ tsp. Fresh dill

Ground black pepper and salt, to taste

2 oz. Finely chopped dill

1 Celery stalk, finely chopped

2 oz. Red onion, chopped

1 tbsp. Salted keto cucumber, chopped

6 Hard-boiled eggs, chopped

Paprika, for garnish

1. Pour some water (about 2.5 cm) into a large saucepan, put 1 tsp. of salt and bring to a boil. Add cauliflower and cook until ready, from 8 to 10 minutes. Drain and set aside in a large bowl.

2. In a small bowl, mix mayonnaise, mustard, dill, a pinch of salt and pepper. Set aside.

3. Crush 4 eggs and add to the cauliflower bowl. Slice the remaining two eggs.

4. Add pickled cucumber, celery, 1/4 teaspoon salt, pepper and red onion. Add all the ingredients to the cauliflower and shake gently.

5. Garnish with the remaining chopped eggs and sprinkle with paprika.

PER SERVING

Calories: 222. Fat: 20 g. Protein: 8 g. Carbs: 2

5. Light Pea and Green Onion Salad

Prep. time: 5 minutes / Cook time: 10 minutes / Serves2

2 oz. Pea

2 tsp. Green onions

½ tsp. Soy sauce

2 tsp. Olive oil

½ tsp. Apple vinegar

½ tsp. Sesame oil

½ tsp. Sesame seeds

Garlic powder, to taste

1. Slice the green onions and peas diagonally.

2. Mix the chopped vegetables with the remaining ingredients

and mix. Cover and refrigerate for 2 hours.

3. Serve with the main course of your choice - grilled chicken, shrimps, salmon, etc.

PER SERVING

Calories: 136. Fat: 14 g. Protein: 2.5 g. Carbs: 3g

6. Keto-Salsa with Avocado and Shrimps

Prep. time: 10 minutes / Cook time: 10 minutes / Serves4

8 oz. Peeled raw shrimp

1 tbsp. Olive oil

1 Lemon (juice)

1 Avocado, diced

1 Tomato, diced

1 Cucumber, diced

1/4 Onion, diced

2 oz. Cilantro, chopped

Salt and black pepper, to taste

1. Season the shrimp with salt and pepper. Put the pan on a medium-high heat and pour olive oil. Once the oil has warmed up, add the shrimp and fry one side for 2-3 minutes, then turn to the other.

2. Remove the shrimps from the pan and put them on a cutting board. Slice and transfer to a large bowl.

3. Squeeze the marinade lemon juice into the bowl. Mix well and let stand for a while.

4. Add pieces of avocado, tomatoes and cucumbers to the bowl.

5. Mix with chopped onion and cilantro. Mix well all together.

PER SERVING

Calories: 283. Fat: 18.8 g. Protein: 18 g. Carbs: 6.2

7. Keto Salad Taco

Prep. time: 10 minutes / Cook time: 20 minutes / Serves4

1 lb. Ground beef from grass-fed meat

1 tsp. Ground cumin

½ tsp. Chili powder

1 tbsp. Garlic powder

½ tbsp. Paprika

Salt and pepper, to taste

4 cup Roman lettuce

1 Tomato

4 oz. Cheddar cheese

4 oz. Cilantro

1 Avocado

4 oz. Favorite salsa

2 small limes

1 cup Cucumber, sliced

1. Heat a large skillet over medium heat and pour in some coconut oil. Add ground beef and all seasonings.

2. Mix well and fry until brown. Remove from heat and cool slightly.

3. Mix roman lettuce, vegetables, cheese and chopped avocado. Top with meat, salsa and a generous portion of lime juice. Mix everything well.

PER SERVING

Calories: 430. Fat: 31 g. Protein: 29 g. Carbs:

CHAPTER FIVE

8. Snacks Quick Keto Bread

Prep. time: 5 minutes / Cook time: 10 minutes / Serves10

2 tbsp. Almond flour

½ tbsp. Coconut flour

1/4 tsp. Baking powder

1 Egg

½ tbsp. Ghee or butter

1 tbsp. Unsweetened milk of your choice

1. Mix all ingredients in a small bowl and whisk until smooth.

2. Grease a glass bowl or microwave dish with butter, ghee or coconut oil.

3. Pour the dough into a mold and place in the microwave at high temperature for 90 seconds.

4. Slice and pour melted butter as desired.

PER SERVING

Calories: 45. Fat: 20 g. Protein: 7 g. Carbs: 3

Note: If you do not have a microwave, try frying the dough in a small amount of butter / coconut oil or ghee.

The same cooking time, the same easy recipe is just a slightly different texture.

9. Energy Keto Bars with Nuts and Seeds

Prep. time: 10 minutes / Cook time: 25 minutes / Serves 8

2 tbsp. Butter or coconut oil

2 fl. oz. Sugar-free

1 tsp. Vanilla extract

8 oz. Almond, chopped

8 oz. Raw macadamia nuts (finely chopped)

4 oz. Pumpkin seed

2 tbsp. Hemp seed

1-2 tsp. Keto sweetener (if necessary)

4 oz. Low sugar chocolate chips

½ tsp. Coconut or butter, or ghee oil

1. Preheat the oven to 350 °F degrees and lay out a baking dish with

parchment paper. Put all the nuts and seeds in a large bowl, and mix.

2. Melt butter or coconut oil with vanilla extract and syrup in a small saucepan over low heat.

3. Pour the hot mixture over the nuts and seeds, and shake well. If necessary, add keto sweetener (erythritol, stevia, etc.)

4. Pour the resulting mass into the prepared baking dish.

5. Bake for about 22-25 minutes until the top turns golden brown. Allow the mixture to cool for at least 45 minutes.

6. Melt the chocolate and 1/2 tsp of coconut oil in the microwave or on the stove.

Pour a mixture of baked nuts and seeds.

7. Put in the freezer for 10-15 minutes. Remove from the mold and cut into 8 pieces.

PER SERVING

Calories: 303. Fat: 29 g. Protein: 8 g. Carbs: 4g

10. Low-Carb Flax Bread

Prep. time: 10 minutes / Cook time: 15 minutes / Serves8

1 oz. Almond flour

1½ Flaxseed

1 tsp. Baking powder

Salt, to taste

½ tsp. Vinegar

4 drops Liquid stevia

3 oz. Raw whisked egg

1 fl. oz. Coconut oil or butter

(melted)

1. Mix together all the dry ingredients, then mix the wet ones.

2. Stir dry ingredients with wet ones.

3. Spread the dough into a lightly oiled form.

4. Bake at 350 °F degrees for 8–10 minutes.

PER SERVING

Calories: 35. Fat: 42 g. Protein: 14 g. Carbs: 6g

11. Keto Mini Pizza

Prep. time: 5 minutes / Cook time: 15 minutes / Serves4

1 oz. Keto mayonnaise

1 tbsp. Raw eggs

2 tsp. Coconut oil, melted

2 tsp. Almond flour

1 tsp. Coconut flour

½ tsp. Psyllium powder

A pinch of baking powder and baking soda

1. Heat the oven to 400 °F degrees.

2. Mix all the ingredients well to form a dough. Make sure there are no lumps in it.

3. Leave the dough to stand for about 5 minutes.

4. Divide the dough into 3-4 small balls, about 2.5 cm in diameter.

5. Lay out a baking sheet with parchment paper. Put dough balls on the parchment and press down on them to make small pizzas.

6. Put the stuffing on the raw dough and bake for 7-9 minutes.

PER SERVING

Calories: 112. Fat: 28 g. Protein: 4 g. Carbs: 2

12. Baked Eggs with Ham and Asparagus

Prep. time: 5 minutes / Cook time: 15 minutes / Serves 2

6 Eggs

6 slices (about 4 oz.) Italian ham

1. Heat the oven to 350 °F degrees.

2. Grease a muffin tray.

3. Lay the ham down and around the hole so as to cover the bottom and sides.

4. Add a few twigs of marjoram.

5. Pour 1 egg into each form.

6. Put in the oven and bake 10 - 12 minutes until cooked.

7. Pull out and allow to cool for a few minutes.

8. Steam the asparagus, then season it with butter.

9. Put all the ingredients on a plate and enjoy.

PER SERVING

Calories: 424. Fat: 33 g. Protein: 30 g. Carbs: 2.5g

13. Eggplant Keto Chips

Prep. time: 5 minutes / Cook time: 20 minutes / Serves 4

2 fl. oz. Olive oil

1 Large eggplant (thinly sliced)

Sal and pepper to taste

1 tsp. Garlic powder

½ tsp. Dry basil

½ tsp. Dried oregano

1. Preheat oven to 350 °F degrees.

2. Add 1/4 cup olive oil and dried spices to a small bowl. Roll the sliced eggplant in oil and spices, and place it on a baking sheet.

3. Bake for about 15-20 minutes, until the chips are evenly fried. Turn them over a couple of times during cooking.

4. Remove from the oven and sprinkle with Parmesan cheese (optional)

PER SERVING

Calories: 60. Fat: 5 g. Protein: 2 g. Carbs: 1

14. Cheese Keto Sticks

Prep. time: 5 minutes / Cook time: 15 minutes / Serves3

3 Mozzarella cheese sticks (cut in half)

4 oz. Almond flour

1 tbsp. Italian seasoning mixes

2 tbsp. Grated parmesan cheese

1 Big egg

Salt, to taste

2 tbsp. Coconut oil

1 tbsp. Chopped parsley

1. Put the cheese in the freezer overnight so that it hardens.

2. Then add coconut oil to a medium sized cast iron skillet and heat it over low to medium heat.

3. Break the egg into a shallow bowl and whisk well. In a separate bowl, mix the almond flour, parmesan cheese and seasonings.

4. Roll cheese sticks in an egg, then dry breading. Put on a wire rack and bake until golden brown on all sides for about 1-2 minutes.

5. Place chopsticks on paper towels to soak up the oil.

6. Serve with low-carb marinara sauce and parsley (optional).

PER SERVING

Calories: 436. Fat: 39 g. Protein: 20 g. Carbs: 5g

15. Lunch Chicken Keto Nuggets

Prep. time: 15 minutes / Cook time: 6 hours / Serves4

1 oz. Whipped egg whites

1 oz. Chicken breast cooked and minced

½ oz. Coconut flour

½ tsp. Baking powder

1 fl. oz. Olive oil

½ oz. Melted butter

1 oz. Fatty 40% cream

Salt, pepper, a pinch of garlic powder, optional

1. Mix shredded chicken with coconut flour, baking powder and seasoning. The mixture should look very dry.

2. Add butter and mix again. Add whipped egg whites and mix until smooth.

3. Pour olive oil into a small non-stick pan. Spread the chicken-egg mixture in small pieces and fry for about 1 minute on each side.

4. Serve with whipped cream, diluted with water, like "milk".

PER SERVING

Calories: 136. Fat: 41 g. Protein: 9 g. Carbs: 2

16. Champignon Keto Burger

Prep. time: 5 minutes / Cook time: 15 minutes / Serves 4

2 Large champignons, without legs

2 tbsp. Olive oil

1 tbsp. Balsamic vinegar

2 Slices of bacon

4 oz. Ground beef

½ tsp. Garlic powder

½ tsp. Onion powder

½ tsp. Worcestershire Sauce

1 Cheddar cheese, slice

1 Slice of tomato

2 oz. Mixed greens or arugula

1 tbsp. Low-sugar ketchup

1. Put the mushroom caps in a bowl or shallow plate, and add

olive oil, balsamic vinegar and half the salt and pepper; marinate for at least 30 minutes.

2. Cook the bacon in a frying pan over medium heat until crisp, turning a couple

of times to fry each side evenly. Set aside.

3. Preheat the oven and turn on the grill function (270 °F degrees). Mix in a bowl ground beef, garlic and onion powder, Worcestershire sauce and the remaining salt and pepper.Form the patties for burgers.

4. Put the caps of champignons and cutlets on the grill, and cook for about 3-4 minutes on each side until they are soft. At the last minute, put the cheese on the cutlets so that it melts.

5. Assemble the hamburger with bacon and the rest of the stuffing between the mushroom caps.

PER SERVING

Calories: 771. Fat: 67 g. Protein: 37 g. Carbs: 4g

17.   Nourishing Beef Soup

Prep. time: 10 minutes / Cook time: 30 minutes / Serves 8

1 lb. Ground beef

5 Slices of bacon

1 tbsp. Olive oil

1 tbsp. Minced garlic

1 cup Chopped celery

1½ cup Bone broth

1 cup Shredded cheddar

2 fl. oz. Fat whipped cream

2 tsp. Psyllium powder

4 oz. Shredded cheddar cheese

½ oz. Chopped green onions

½ cup Sour cream

1. Fry the bacon over medium heat, then place it on paper towels to remove excess fat. Then crush it into pieces.

2. Then fry the ground beef over medium heat. After cooking, drain the fat and transfer the minced meat to a bowl.

3. In the same pan, melt butter over medium heat. Add

chopped garlic and fry until fragrant.

4. Add the celery and cook until slightly softened, about 5 minutes.

5. Put the ground beef in the pan. Add beef broth, cheddar, rich whipped cream, sautéed celery with garlic, bacon, salt and pepper. Cook for 20 minutes, stirring occasionally.

6. To obtain the desired thickness, add psyllium powder.

7. Pour into portions and add a side dish in the form of cheese, green onions and sour cream (optional).

PER SERVING

Calories: 349. Fat: 27 g. Protein: 23 g. Carbs: 3g

18.   Keto Cheeseburger with Bacon

Prep. time: 10 minutes / Cook time: 30 minutes / Serves2

For the dough:

8 oz. Mozzarella, shredded

4 oz. Almond flour

1 tbsp. Cream cheese

For filling:

5 oz. Ground beef

1 Slice of cheddar cheese, cut

into quarters

1 tsp. Mustard

4 Bacon, slices

1 Whisked egg

1 tsp. Sesame

1 tsp. Olive oil

Salad Leaves for Garnish

(Optional)

1. Preheat oven to 420 °F degrees.

2. Mix mozzarella, almond flour and cream cheese in a bowl. Heat the mixture in the microwave for 1 minute, mix and re-set in the microwave for 1 minute.

3. Form two patties from ground beef. Put on the cutting board.

4. strips of bacon crosswise, cutlet on top, then cheddar slices, the second cutlet, and then wrap all the bacon.

4. Heat the olive oil in a frying pan over medium heat, put the patties in bacon and fry for 3 minutes on each side.

5. Roll the dough between 2 sheets of parchment paper.

Remove the top sheet and place mustard in the center of the dough. On top, put the patty in bacon and wrap the dough.

6. Put the burger in the oven, coat with beaten egg, sprinkle with sesame seeds and bake for 15-20 minutes or until golden brown.

7. Take out and serve with sheets of greens.

PER SERVING

Calories: 411. Fat: 32 g. Protein: 27 g.
Carbs: 3g

19. Spicy Keto Soup with Mushrooms

Prep. time: 10 minutes / Cook time: 30 minutes / Serves 4

1 tbsp. Olive oil

1 Onion (thinly sliced)

1 tbsp. Fresh grated ginger

3 Garlic, cloves (finely chopped)

1 tsp. Chile

1 tbsp. Fish sauce

2 fl. oz. Soy sauce

2 fl. oz. Rice vinegar

4 oz. Mushrooms (thinly sliced)

4 Hard boiled eggs

2-3 packets of shirataki noodles

5 cup Bone broth

1. Pour oil into a large saucepan and put on medium heat.

Add the onion and cook for 2-3 minutes until soft.

2. Add the remaining ingredients to the pan (except eggs and noodles). Cook over low heat for 20-30 minutes.

3. Remove the noodles from the package and rinse well undermcold water.

4. Add seasoning to the broth and mix with noodles.

5. Pour the broth into portions. Add hard-boiled eggs, chopped chicken or beef, cilantro, sesame seeds, chopped

green onions and chili sauce (all optional).

PER SERVING

Calories: 103. Fat: 13 g. Protein: 12 g. Carbs: 7g

20. Greek Keto Moussaka

Prep. time: 10 minutes / Cook time: 30 minutes / Serves 4

For filling:

½ Chopped eggplant

10 oz. Minced chicken

3 tbsp. Marinara sauce

1 Minced garlic

½ Chopped onion

1 tsp. Dried oregano

1 tsp. Paprika

½ tsp. Ground cinnamon

2 tbsp. Olive oil

For the sauce:

3 tbsp. Heavy cream

3 tbsp. Cream cheese

3 oz. Crushed cheddar cheese

1 Minced garlic

1. Lay out a foil baking sheet. Cut the eggplants, put them on a baking sheet and pour olive oil. Bake the eggplants for 5 minutes or until golden brown.

2. Heat olive oil in a frying pan, add chopped onion, chopped

garlic and fry until soft. Add chopped chicken and seasonings, and fry until the meat is cooked. Add the marinara sauce, mix and cook for another 3 minutes.

3. Mix half the crushed cheddar cheese, cream cheese, heavy cream, garlic and salt in a saucepan, and cook on low heat until the cheese is melted and the sauce becomes thick and uniform.

4. Preheat oven to 400 °F degrees. Place the pieces of fried eggplant on a baking sheet, top the chicken mixture, pour the sauce, sprinkle with the remaining cheese and bake for 20 minutes.

5. Let the dish stand for 5 minutes before serving. May be served with green salad or greens.

PER SERVING

Calories: 358. Fat: 29 g. Protein: 20 g. Carbs: 4g

21. Almond Pancakes with Shrimp and Cheese

Prep. time: 10 minutes / Cook time: 10 minutes / Serves 8

1 lb. Shrimp cooked and chopped

2 oz. Almond flour

1 Whisked egg

2 oz. Mozzarella, shredded

3 tbsp. Parmesan cheese, grated

1 tbsp. Fresh dill, chopped

1½ tbsp. Olive or coconut oil, for frying

Salt and pepper, to taste

1. Mix the shrimp, egg, almond flour, cheese, dill and seasonings in a bowl and mix well until smooth.

2. Using a tablespoon to form pancakes. The size of each depends on your taste.

3. Heat the oil in a pan over medium heat and fry pancakes for 3-4 minutes on each side or until cooked.

4. Put on a plate and serve with herbs and aioli, or any other sauce of your choice.

PER SERVING

Calories: 364. Fat: 21 g. Protein: 41 g. Carbs: 2g

Dinner

22.   Baked Halibut Cheese Breaded

Prep. time: 10 minutes / Cook time: 15 minutes / Serves 6

2 lb. Halibut (about 6 fillets)

1 tbsp. Butter

3 tbsp. Grated parmesan cheese

1 tbsp. Bread crumbs

2 tsp. Garlic powder

1 tbsp. Dried parsley

Salt and pepper, to taste

1. Preheat the oven to 400 °F degrees. Mix all ingredients thoroughly in a bowl, except the plate.

2. Dry the fish fillets with a paper towel and place each piece on a greased buttered parchment tray.

3. Spread the cheese mixture into pieces of fish so that it covers its top.

4. Bake the fish for 10-12 minutes (turn the baking tray at least once).

5. Increase heat for 2–3 minutes until the top is golden brown.

Check readiness with a fork.

PER SERVING

Calories: 330. Fat: 30 g. Protein: 13 g. Carbs: 2g

23. Tandoori Chicken Legs

Prep. time: 10 minutes / Cook time: 25 minutes / Serves 2

2 Whole chicken legs

4 fl. oz. Fatty Greek yogurt

2 tbsp. Olive oil

½ tsp. Cumin

½ tsp. Turmeric

½ tsp. Coriander

1/4 tsp. Cardamom

½ tsp. Cayenne pepper

1 tsp. Paprika

Pinch of Nutmeg

1 Minced garlic clove

½ tsp. Fresh ginger

2 tbsp. Lime juice

Salt and pepper, to taste

1. Heat olive oil in a small frying pan over medium heat. Add cumin, turmeric, coriander, cardamom, cayenne pepper, paprika and a pinch of nutmeg. Heat the spices, then remove from heat and cool.

2. Mix in a bowl yogurt with spiced oil, lime juice, ginger, chopped garlic, salt and pepper.

3. Make 3-4 deep cuts on each leg and pour spicy yogurt into them.
Cover and refrigerate for 6 hours.

4. Lubricate the rack for frying olive oil and place on a baking sheet. Put the chicken on the rack and fry for 5 minutes on each side.

5. Set the oven to 360 °F degrees and continue cooking for 25 minutes.

6. Serve with cauliflower rice.

PER SERVING

Calories: 372. Fat: 28 g. Protein: 30 g. Carbs: 2g

24. Baked Eggplant with Cheese

Prep. time: 15 minutes / Cook time: 60 minutes / Serves 4

1 Large eggplant, sliced

1 Big egg

½ cup Parmesan cheese, grated

¼ cup Pork dough

½ tbsp. Italian seasoning

1 cup low-sugar tomato sauce

½ cup Mozzarella, shredded

4 tbsp. Butter

1. Preheat oven to 400 °F degrees. Put the sliced eggplant on a baking sheet lined with a paper towel and sprinkle with salt on both sides. Let stand for at least 30 minutes so that all the water comes out of the eggplant.

2. Mix the chopped pork cracklings, parmesan cheese and Italian seasoning in a shallow dish. Set aside.

3. In a separate small plate, beat an egg.

4. Melt the butter and grease the baking dish with it.

5. Dip each piece of eggplant in a beaten egg, and then in a mixture of parmesan and cracklings, covering each side with crumbs.

6. Place the eggplants in a baking dish and bake for 20minutes. Turn the eggplant slices over and bake for another 20 minutes or until golden brown.

7. Top with tomato sauce and sprinkle with chopped mozzarella.

8. Return the mold to the oven for another 5 minutes, or until the cheese has melted.

PER SERVING

Calories: 376. Fat: 28 g. Protein: 19 g. Carbs: 7g

25. Shrimp and Zucchini with Alfredo Sauce

Prep. time: 5 minutes / Cook time: 15 minutes / Serves 6

8 oz. Shrimp, peeled

2 tbsp. Butter

½ tsp Minced garlic

1 tbsp. Fresh lemon juice

2 Zucchini

2 oz. Heavy cream

3 oz. Parmesan cheese

Salt and pepper to taste

1. Use the scoop to make zucchini noodles.

2. Heat the butter in a frying pan, add the chopped garlic, red pepper and fry for 1 minute, stirring constantly.

3. Add shrimp and simmer for about 3 minutes. Add salt and pepper, remove from pan and set aside.

4. In the same pan (with shrimp juice), add heavy cream, lemon juice, parmesan, and cook for 2 minutes.

5. Add the noodles from zucchini and cook another 2 minutes, stirring occasionally.

6. Put the shrimp back in the pan and mix well.

7. If necessary, add salt and pepper, garnish with parmesan and chopped parsley (optional) and serve immediately.

PER SERVING

Calories: 404. Fat: 28 g. Protein: 32 g. Carbs: 5g

26. Chicken Breasts in a Garlic-Cream Sauce

Prep. time: 10 minutes / Cook time: 25 minutes / Serves 4

For chicken:

2 Chicken breasts

1 tbsp. Lemon juice

1/4 tsp. Chili powder

1 tsp. Fresh grated ginger

1 Minced garlic

½ tsp. Coriander powder

½ tsp. Turmeric

1 oz. Butter

For the sauce:

4 oz. Heavy cream

3 tbsp. Crushed tomatoes

4 fl. oz. Chicken broth

1 Onion, diced

1 Garlic clove, minced

1/4 tsp. Chili powder

1 tsp. Fresh grated ginger

1/4 tsp. Cinnamon

1. Cut the chicken breasts into small pieces then mix them in a bowl with lemon juice, chili powder, grated ginger, chopped garlic, coriander powder, turmeric, salt and pepper.

2. Heat 2 tablespoons of butter in a frying pan over medium heat, then add the onions and garlic, and simmer for 2 minutes or until fragrant.

3. Add chicken pieces and cook for 4-5 minutes. When the chicken is white, add heavy cream, chicken broth, chopped

tomatoes, seasonings and mix well. Bring to a boil, then reduce the heat to minimum, cover and simmer for 6-7 minutes.

4. If you like sauce thicker - remove the lid and simmer it to the desired consistency.

5. Serve with steamed broccoli or any other low-carb product to your taste.

PER SERVING

Calories: 319. Fat: 21 g. Protein: 27 g. Carbs: 3.9g

27. Salmon Fillet with Cream Sauce

Prep. time: 10 minutes / Cook time: 15 minutes / Serves 3

2 tbsp. Olive oil

3 Salmon fillets

2 Garlic cloves, minced

1 cup Heavy whipped cream

1 oz. Cream cheese

2 tbsp. Capers

1 tbsp. Lemon juice

2 tsp. Fresh dill

2 tbsp. Parmesan cheese, grated

1. Place a large frying pan over medium heat and heat the olive oil. Once the pan is hot, add the salmon fillet, frying each side for about five minutes.

2. As soon as the salmon is cooked, remove it from the pan and set aside.

3. In the same pan, roast the chopped garlic over medium heat to a flavorful state.

4. Add heavy cream, cream cheese, lemon juice and capers.

5. Bring the mixture to a light boil, stirring often to thicken.

6. As soon as the sauce begins to thicken, put the salmon back in the pan and cover it with creamy sauce.

7. Reduce heat to medium-low - just to warm the fillet.

8. Garnish with fresh dill and grated Parmesan cheese.

PER SERVING

Calories: 494. Fat: 31 g. Protein: 53 g. Carbs: 2.5g

28. Beef Casserole with Cabbage and Cheese

Prep. time: 15 minutes / Cook time: 30 minutes / Serves 8

1 tbsp. Worcestershire Sauce

1 cup Shredded cracklings

1 Big egg

2 cup Cheddar cheese, grated

2 lb. Cauliflower

8 oz. Softened cream cheese

1 lb. Grounded beef

½ Onion, diced

5 oz. Bacon

Salt and pepper, to taste

Extra side dish: chopped onion

1. Cut the bacon, and fry it in a hot frying pan. Place it on a paper towel to absorb excess fat. Remove most of the fat from the pan, you will need only a few tablespoons.

2. Fry the onions in bacon fat until it turned to golden brown.

3. Add grounded beef and fry well. Add the Worcestershire sauce and, if necessary, seasonings.
Transfer the mixture to a large bowl.

4. Get a separate bowl, mix in the cabbage and cream cheese then whisk everything together using a hand mixer or blender.
The consistency of everything should be like mashed potatoes. If necessary, add seasoning.

5. Add chopped bacon and egg to beef mixture and mix well.

6. Place the grounded beef on the bottom of the baking dish and place the cauliflower puree on top.

7. Sprinkle casserole with chopped cheddar cheese and bacon.

8. Bake in the oven at 400 °F for 30 minutes.

9. If you want, sprinkle the finished dish with chopped onion.

PER SERVING

Calories: 443. Fat: 35 g. Protein: 24 g. Carbs: 5.4g

29. Creamy Spinach

Prep. time: 10 minutes / Cook time: 20 minutes / Serves 4

1 Onion, diced

2 Garlic cloves, minced

9 oz. Fresh spinach

2 tbsp. Butter

2 tbsp. Olive oil

2 fl. oz. Cream cheese

2 fl. oz. Heavy cream

1. Heat the cream and olive oil in a frying pan at medium-high temperature.

2. Add garlic and onions, and stir continuously for 2-3 minutes until soft.

3. Add the spinach (handful at a time) and fry until it withers.

Put in a fine strainer and squeeze the liquid.

4. Return the spinach to the pan, season with pepper and salt then add the heavy cream. Cook until there are bubbles in the cream.

5. Mix with cream cheese until it is completely melted, and the mixture is thick and bubbly. Remove from heat and serve.

PER SERVING

Calories: 277. Fat: 21 g. Protein: 9 g. Carbs: 7g

30. Fried Cod with Tomato Sauce

Prep. time: 10 minutes / Cook time: 20 minutes / Serves 4

A fish:

1 tbsp. Olive oil

Salt and pepper, to taste

1 lb. (4 fillets) Cod

1 tbsp. Butter

Tomato sauce:

3 tbsp. Warm water

8 oz. Butter

2 tbsp. Tomato paste

3 Large egg yolks

2 tbsp. Fresh lemon juice

For fish:

1. Season the fillets on both sides. Note that the salt must be added at the last minute, before cooking, so as not to burn the fish.

2. Pour olive oil beneath the bottom of the anti-grate pan and turn on medium heat. Add butter. When they begin to sizzle, add cod fillet and fry for two or three minutes, then turn it over to the other side.

3. Tilt the pan, collect the oil with a spoon and dip the fish in it. Continue cooking for another two or three minutes.

Tomato sauce:

1. Melt the butter.

2. Boil egg yolks and warm water (1 tablespoon of water for each egg yolk) for two minutes until thick and creamy.

3. When the yolks have reached the desired consistency remove them from the heat. Begin to beat them, slowly pour in the butter. Beat until smooth.

4. Season with salt and pepper. You can add herbs if you so desire.

5. Add tomato paste and mix together.

6. Add lemon juice and adjust the consistency with a little warm water to dilute the sauce slightly.

PER SERVING

Calories: 589. Fat: 56 g. Protein: 20 g. Carbs: 2g

31.   Braised Beef in Orange Sauce

Prep. time: 10 minutes / Cook time: 90 minutes / Serves 6

3 tbsp. Coconut oil

1 Onion

Peel and juice of 1 orange

2 tbsp. Apple vinegar

1 tbsp. Fresh thyme

2 tsp. Erythritol

2 lb. Beef

3 cups Beef broth

2½ tsp. Garlic, chopped

2 tsp. Ground cinnamon

1 tsp. Soy sauce

Rosemary, sage, bay leaf, salt, pepper, to taste

1. Cut vegetables and meat into cubes. Squeeze orange juice and rub it in zest.

2. Heat up coconut oil in a cast iron skillet.

3. Add seasoned meat (salt + pepper) to the pan in batches. Do not overfill the pan.

4. Fry it until brown and remove from the pan.

5. When your beef is ready, add vegetables to the pan. Cook for 1-2 minutes.

6. Add orange juice and then put all the other ingredients in the pan, with the exception of rosemary, sage and thyme.

7. Cook for 30 seconds, and then add all other ingredients.

8. Stew for 3 hours.

9. Open the pan and add the remaining spices. Allow it to cook for 1-2 hours.

PER SERVING

Calories: 337. Fat: 14 g. Protein:42 g. Carbs: 5g

32. Meatloaf

Prep. time: 10 minutes / Cook time: 60 minutes / Serves 8

6 slices Cheddar cheese

½ cup Spinach

2 oz. Sliced onions

2 oz. Green onions, chopped

1 lb. Grounded beef

½ tsp. Garlic powder

½ tsp. Cumin

¼ cup Mushrooms

1.Mix up the meat with salt, pepper, garlic and cumin.

2.Put the stuffing in the form, create in the middle a place for the filling.

3. Put cheese on the bottom of the roll.

4. Add onions, spinach and mushrooms.

5. Use the remaining meat to cover the top with spinach and mushrooms as a cover.

6. Bake at 370 °F for one hour.

PER SERVING

Calories: 248. Fat: 21 g. Protein: 15 g. Carbs: 2g

33. Keto Chili

Prep. time: 10 minutes / Cook time: 30 minutes / Serves 6

2 lb. Young beef

2 Green bell peppers

1 Onion

1 tsp. Garlic powder

1 tbsp. Olive oil

1 tbsp. Cumin

1½ tbsp. Chili powder

2 tsp. Cayenne pepper

8 oz. Spinach

1 cup Tomato sauce

2 oz. Parmesan cheese

Salt and pepper, to taste

1. Slice the onions and peppers and season with salt and simmer in olive oil at medium high temperature, stirring occasionally. When the vegetables are ready, reduce the heat to minimum.

2. Fry the beef until brown. season with salt, pepper and spices.

3. When the beef is fried, add the spinach. Cook for 2-3 minutes, then mix well.

4. Add tomato sauce, mix well, and then reduce the heat to medium-low and cook for 10 minutes.

5. Add Parmesan cheese and mix everything together.

Then add the vegetables and mix again. Cook for a few minutes.

PER SERVING

Calories: 404. Fat: 27 g. Protein: 31 g. Carbs: 5g

34. Beef Croquettes with Sausage and Cheese

Prep. time: 10 minutes / Cook time: 30 minutes / Serves12

1 cup Cheddar cheese

2 Large eggs

1 lb. Minced beef

1 Chorizo sausage

1 tsp. Cumin

8 fl. oz. Tomato sauce

3 oz. Shredded pork skins

1 tsp. Chili

1. Preheat oven to 380 °F degrees.

2. Cut the sausage into smaller pieces and mix well with the beef.

3. Add pork skins, spices, cheese and eggs.

4. Mix up everything together until you can form the meatballs.

5. Put them on a baking tray with a baking sheet.

6. Bake in the oven for 30-35 minutes.

7. Top up with tomato sauce.

PER SERVING

Calories: 142. Fat: 12 g. Protein: 7 g. Carbs: 1g

35. Eggplant with Bacon

Prep. time: 10 minutes / Cook time: 20 minutes / Serves 6

2 Garlic cloves, grated

1 lb. Bacon

1 lb. Eggplant

1 tbsp. White wine

1 cup Heavy whipped cream

2 tbsp. Butter

1 tbsp. Lemon juice

1 cup Parmesan cheese, shredded

1. Slice the bacon and fry in a large frying pan over a medium heat.

2. When the bacon is crispy, pull it out of the pan and place it on a paper towel. Drain all the fat.

3. Peel and slice the eggplant. Cook it in bacon fat until is softens.

4. As cooking progresses, the eggplant will absorb all the fat.

Clean the center of the place and pour 2 tablespoons of oil into it. Stir everything so that the eggplants are covered in melted butter, then add the grated garlic.

5. Pour a cup of heavy whipped cream into the pan.

Then add white wine and lemon juice.

6. Add a cup of shredded Parmesan cheese and mix.

7. Mix up everything with about half the bacon.

8. Serve with the remaining bacon, laid out on top.

You can also chop fresh basil from above.

PER SERVING

Calories: 564. Fat: 51 g. Protein: 16 g. Carbs: 6g

Desserts

36.   Cheesecake Keto-Cupcakes

Prep. time: 10 minutes / Cook time: 15 minutes / Serves12

2 oz. Butter, melted

8 fl. oz. Soft cream cheese

2 Eggs

4 oz. Almond flour

6 oz. Granulated keto sweetener

1 tsp. Vanilla extract

1. Heat the oven to 350 °F degrees. Arrange the parchment 12molds for muffins.

2. Mix up together butter and almond flour, then spread the mixture with a

spoon over the forms and slightly push it inside.

3. Combine cream cheese, eggs, sweetener and vanilla extract with in a mixer until smooth. Spread the spoon on top of the dough in the tins.

4. Bake in a preheated oven for 15 to 17 minutes.

5. Before serving, cupcakes should stand in the refrigerator for about 8 hours.

PER SERVING

Calories: 204. Fat: 21 g. Protein: 4.9 g. Carbs: 2g

37. Chocolates with Berries

Prep. time: 10 minutes / Cook time: 15 minutes / Serves12

1 tbsp. Erythritol or xylitol

1 tbsp. Liquid coconut oil

2 tbsp. Cocoa butter

4 tbsp. Solid coconut oil

2 tbsp. Cocoa powder

1 cup Fresh berries mix

Optional: grated unsweetened coconut or raw chopped nuts

1. Mix up solid coconut oil, cocoa butter, liquid coconut oil, salt,
cocoa powder and sweetener to taste in a saucepan, then stir over low heat until completely dissolved.

2. Pour the chocolate mixture into the silicone tray for at least 12 forms.

Sprinkle berries evenly (along with any other additives, if used).

3. Place the tray in the fridge for about 15 minutes.

4. Store left overs in a refrigerator in a closed container.

PER SERVING

Calories: 61. Fat: 6 g. Protein: 1 g. Carbs: 2g

38.   Keto Cookies with Raspberry Jam

Prep. time: 10 minutes / Cook time: 15 minutes / Serves12

2 cup Almond flour

2 oz. Erythritol or other keto friendly sweetener

1 tsp. Vanilla extract

1 Egg

1/4 tsp Xanthan gum

½ tsp. Baking powder

4 oz. Soft butter

3 tbsp. Raspberry jam / sugar free jam

1. Preheat the oven to 370 °F degrees and place a baking sheet with parchment paper.

2. Mix up flour, xanthan gum, baking powder and salt in a small bowl. Put aside.

3. Get a separate bowl, beat the butter and sweetener until the mass becomes airy.

4. Add egg and vanilla extract.

5. Add the flour mixture and mix well.

6. Share the dough into 12 balls and place on the prepared baking sheet.

7. Click on the center of each ball to make a cookie.

In the center of each place 1/2 tsp. of jam.

8. Bake cookies for 10–12 minutes, until the edges are light golden brown.

9. Allow to cool until the jam hardens.

PER SERVING

Calories: 168. Fat: 16 g. Protein: 4 g. Carbs: 2g

39. Chocolate Brownie in a Mug

Prep. time: 5 minutes / Cook time: 10 minutes / Serves 12

1 tbsp. Butter or coconut oil

½ tsp. Vanilla extract

1 Big egg

2 tbsp. Almond flour

½ tsp. Baking powder

2 tbsp. Unsweetened cocoa powder

1 tbsp. Stevia or any keto-friendly sweetener of your choice

1. Oil one large cup or two small shapes. Put aside.

2. Mix all ingredients to a small bowl and mix with a small whisk until smooth.

3. Pour the dough into the prepared form and place in the microwave for about 1 minute (two servings) or 75 seconds per serving in a mug.

PER SERVING

Calories: 140. Fat: 9 g. Protein: 11 g. Carbs: 3g

40. Lemon Blueberry Keto-Cakes

Prep. time: 10 minutes / Cook time: 20 minutes / Serves12

Dough:

4 Eggs

3/4 cup Fatty coconut milk

1 tsp. Baking powder

½ tsp. Xanthan gum

3/4 cup Fresh blueberries

1/8 tsp. Pink Himalayan salt

1 tsp. Pure vanilla extract

½ cup Coconut flour

1½ tbsp. Xylitol

3 tbsp. Herbal unsalted butter, melted

Lemon icing:

1 Lemon, juice and zest

5 tbsp. Powdered (non-granular) stevia or xylitol

1. Preheat the oven to 370 °F degrees.

2. In a large bowl, mix the eggs, coconut milk and vanilla.

3. Add coconut flour, xylitol, baking powder, xanthan gum and salt, and beat well. Add melted butter and mix again.

4. Carefully add fresh blueberries.

5. Fill 12 cupcakes with dough, about half.

6. Place a baking tray with forms on the central grid of the oven and bake for about 20 minutes.

7. Remove from oven and cool.

8. Mix lemon juice with powdered sweetener and pour each cupcake with a small amount of icing.

Garnish with fresh lemon peel.

PER SERVING

Calories: 136. Fat: 7 g. Protein: 9 g. Carbs: 6g

41. Chocolate Keto Fudge

Prep. time: 5 minutes / Cook time: 10 minutes / Serves12

2 oz. Unsweetened cocoa powder

3 tbsp. Keto sweetener

½ cup Almond oil

½ cup Coconut oil

1 tsp. Vanilla extract

2 oz. Walnuts (optional)

1. Combine coconut and almond oil, and cocoa powder in a blender, and beat until smooth.

2. Add vanilla, sweetener and salt. If desired, add walnuts or other ingredients to your taste.

3. Pour the mixture into a baking dish lined with parchment paper. Put it in the fridge until it is completely cool, then pull it out and cut it into 16 small squares.

Note:

You can try to add the following toppings:

Low carb chocolate crumb

Some peanut butter

Cream cheese

Sea salt

A few drops of peppermint oil

PER SERVING

Calories: 137. Fat: 13 g. Protein: 3 g. Carbs: 2g

42. Cheesecake Mint

Prep. time: 10 minutes / Cook time: 15 minutes / Serves 64

1 lb. Soft cream cheese

15 Whole mint leaves

2 fl. oz cup Heavy cream

1½ cup Almond flour

2½ cup Powdered erythritol

5 tbsp. Melted butter

6 oz. Low-carb black chocolate

1/4 tsp. Mint extract.

1. Preheat the oven to 176 degrees.

2. Place a square baking sheet with parchment paper.

3. In a large bowl, mix the almond flour and half a cup of erythritol.

4. Pour the melted butter into the bowl and mix the ingredients until the dough is formed.

5. Put the dough on a baking sheet and bake for 8 minutes or until light brown.

6. Remove the pan from the oven and cool.

7. Make the filling, whipping cream cheese and remaining erythritol with a mixer until smooth.

8. Put mint leaves and heavy cream in a food processor and blend until smooth.

9. Add the mint mixture to the cream cheese filling and mix well.

10. Put the stuffing on the dough in a baking sheet, then put it in the freezer for 3 hours.

11. Take out the cheesecake from the pan, cut into 64 squares and put it back in the freezer.

12. Melt the chocolate in the microwave, stirring often, until it becomes liquid.

13. Add mint extract, then dip or sprinkle each piece of cheese cake with mint chocolate and let it cool.

PER SERVING

Calories: 121. Fat: 12 g. Protein: 3 g. Carbs: 2g

43. Staples Homemade Keto Mayo

Prep. time: 5 minutes / Cook time: 10 minutes / Serves12

6 fl. oz. Olive oil

4 fl. oz. Coconut oil

1 Egg

2 Egg yolks

1 tsp. Dijon mustard

Pinch of salt and smoked paprika

3 drops Liquid stevia

1. Start by adding oils to the blender bowl to measure them.
Make sure your coconut oil is not hot.

2. Add all other ingredients.

3. Start mixing without lifting the blender.

4. Continue mixing by holding the blender at the bottom of the container.

5. Move the blender up and down until the mayonnaise is fully emulsified.

6. Put mayonnaise in a glass jar with a lid and place in the refrigerator.

If you are using whey, leave on a rack for 7hours, then refrigerate.

NOTE:

If you do not have a dip blender, put all ingredients, except butter, in your blender or food processor, and turn it on. Very carefully and very slowly start adding oil. As the mayonnaise begins to emulsify, you can start adding oil a little faster, until you reach a steady stream.

PER SERVING (1 tbsp.)

Calories: 130. Fat: 14 g. Protein: 1 g. Carbs: 0.5g

44. Homemade Sambal Sauce

Prep. time: 5 minutes / Cook time: 30 minutes / Serves10

1 Onion

2 tsp. Chili peppers, dried

3 tbsp. Low-sugar ketchup

2 tbsp. Coconut oil

Salt, to taste

1. Cut the onion and mix until smooth. Set aside.

2. Cut the dried chilies and remove the seeds. Boil the peppers for about 30 minutes or until soft. Then turn the pepper into a paste.

3. In a heated frying pan, melt coconut oil. Then add all the ingredients and mix thoroughly.

PER SERVING (1 tbsp.)

Calories: 36. Fat: 3 g. Protein: 0.5 g. Carbs: 1.5g

45. Low Carb Ketchup

Prep. time: 5 minutes / Cook time: 5 minutes / Serves10

3/4 cup Tomato paste

2 tbsp. Apple cider vinegar

2 tsp. Keto sweetener

Pinch of salt

1 tsp. Garlic powder

3/4 tsp. Onion powder

Pinch of Cayenne Pepper

1 cup Water

1. Add all the ingredients to a large bowl and whisk well.

2. Adjust the salt and sweetener to taste.

PER SERVING (1 tbsp.)

Calories: 20. Fat: 0 g. Protein: 1 g. Carbs: 2g

46. Dutch Keto Sauce

Prep. time: 5 minutes / Cook time: 5 minutes / Serves10

6 Egg yolks

1 drop Worcestershire sauce

1 drop Low carb hot sauce

1 Lemon, juice

Pinch of salt and ground black pepper

8 oz. Butter

NOTE:

The key to success is to make sure your butter is hot enough to lightly cook eggs. It is imperative that you add the oil immediately after removing it from the microwave.

1. Put the first 5 ingredients in a blender. Heat the butter in the microwave (cover with a paper towel so that it does not splash) for 2-3 minutes.

2. Set the blender to low speed and quickly pour the oil through the top of the blender. Beat about 10-15 seconds until smooth.

PER SERVING (serve for 10 oz.)

Calories: 120. Fat: 12 g. Protein: 2 g. Carbs: 1g

47.   Tapenade Keto Sauce

Prep. time: 5 minutes / Cook time: 5 minutes / Serves 8

1 cup Black olives in brine

1 oz. Capers

4 fl. oz. Mix Olive and Avocado oils

2 Garlic, cloves

3 tbsp. Lemon juice

2 tsp. Apple cider vinegar

1 cup Fresh basil

1 cup Fresh parsley

½ tsp. Black pepper

1. Put all the ingredients in a blender or food processor, and beat at low speed until completely homogeneous.

2. Pour into dishes and store in the refrigerator for up to 1week.

PER SERVING

Calories: 134. Fat: 14 g. Protein: 1 g. Carbs: 2g

48. Meat in Keto Sauce

Prep. time: 5 minutes / Cook time: 5 minutes / Serves 8

1 Lemon juice

3 tbsp. Red wine vinegar

2 tsp. Crushed red pepper

Pinch of salt and black pepper

¼ cup Olive oil

1 Shallot

4 Garlic, cloves

½ cup Cilantro

½ cup Parsley

1. Mix all ingredients except olive oil in a
food processor.

Continuing to beat, pour the oil through
the top of a continuous stream.

2. Season to taste and add more oil and
/ or a couple of tablespoons of water, if
necessary, so that the sauce is more
fluid.

PER SERVING

Calories: 46. Fat: 4 g. Protein: 1 g.
Carbs: 1g

49. Quick Pickled Keto Vegetables

Prep. time: 5 minutes / Cook time: 5 minutes / Serves10

1½ tbsp. Pink Himalayan salt

Optional: 1/4 tsp. granulated stevia

1½ cup Filtered water

1½ cup Apple cider vinegar

Suggested vegetables for quick pickling:

½ cup thinly sliced cucumber

½ cup thinly sliced red onion

6 small whole carrots

½ Asparagus, with cut ends

1. In a small saucepan over medium heat, mix all the ingredients for the brine. Heat the liquid to a gentle boil

until the salt and sweetener dissolve (about 2 minutes).

2. Spread the vegetables into the jars and carefully fill them with brine. Allow the jars to cool, then close the lids and store in the refrigerator (up to 2 months).

PER SERVING

Calories: 10. Fat: 0.1 g. Protein: 0.1 g. Carbs: 2g

GUIDANCE ON GOING OUT TO EAT

It is not so hard to convert many of the eatery menus into dishes that are reasonable for keto-diets. Here are couple of tips on how to make it simplier. Most restaurants offer quality meat and fish dishes. Order them, and request from them to replace the high-carb side dish with vegetables.

Egg dishes for instance scrambled eggs or bacon and eggs are also great.

Another great alternative is a burger without a bun. You can simply not eat bread.

In Mexican eateries, you can enjoy meat dishes with a satisfied portion of cheddar cheese, salsa and guacamole sauces and sour cream.

NOTE: When eating out, choose meat, fish or egg dishes. And order an extra portion of vegetables.

CONCLUSION

At first it may be hard to adhere to Keto Diet. However, the popularity of "clean" food is becoming wider, which makes it simpler to find high-quality low-carb foods.

Take a simple and strict path. The best results can be achieved only by those who carefully restrict the intake of carbs. In the first month try very well to bring the level of carbs consumed as low as possible. Remove from your diet all extra sugar and artificial sweeteners such as diet soda. Restricting them from your diet significantly will help you to reduce sugar cravings.

Drink water and renew electrolytes. The majority of the Keto diet common problems are caused by dehydration and lack of electrolytes. When you begin a keto diet (or if you have been sticking to it for a long time), make sure you drink enough water always, add multivitamin to your diet. If you still encounter side effects, make an order for electrolytes as a separate supplement.

Maintain a nutrition diary. To go beyond the acceptable carbohydrate level is very easy. Unseen and hidden carbs are found in almost every product you consume. Keeping records of what you eat will assist you to control the amount of net carbs consumed and feel responsible for your diet.

The Keto or ketogenic diet is a low-carb, high-fat diet. It lowers blood sugar and insulin levels, changes metabolism from carbohydrates to fats and ketones.
I am very glad that you purchased my book. I am sure that in this book you will find everything that you need to achieve your weight loss goals and it will become easier and more enjoyable. If you enjoy reading this book Please kindly leave a sweet review on this site with 5 star rating. I will really appreciate it.
Thank you.

Intermittent Fasting

What Is Intermittent Fasting?

Intermittent fasting (IF) should not be mistaken for a diet. It is more of a eating regimen where you eat your food during an eating window and stay away from food consumption during the fasting window. You fast *meaning stay away from food or eat no calories* for 14-to-20 hours followed by a shorter 4-to-10 hour period where you eat all the calories you need to eat to lose weight and then…

You keep repeating that 24 hour cycle of fasting for 14-to-20 hours followed by 4-to-10 hours of feasting until you have reached your desired weight loss goal. Before I give you more tip on the most proficient method to use intermittent fasting with your current diet plan to burn more fat faster than you think.

5 reasons Intermittent Fasting burns fat faster than the average diet

1. Intermittent fasting forces your body to burn more fat

After you eat any food your blood sugar rises and your blood sugar (*alongside with the stored carbs/glycogen in your body*) is the calories or energy that your body uses *or burns* to keep you alive, working properly and to do all your day to day activities however...

Intermittent fasting powers your body to burn more body fat.

When you fast or not eat anything for certain periods of time your blood sugar become lower, the amount of carbs stored in your body gets lower and when this occur your body has no choice than to utilize your body fat as the main source of energy to keep you alive, functioning properly and to do all your daily activities and technically.

Your body fat is the accumulation of all the surplus calories you overate so every time you consume excess food; your body takes those accumulated excess calories, stores it as body fat and utilize it as a backup source of energy when you create a energy or calories deficiency from more exercise or eating less (like in any normal weight reduction plan) However your body is likewise forced to mostly only burn body fat **(or cause you to lose weight)** when there is very little blood sugar or carbs left to burn when you fast for 14+ hours.

The less glucose you have in your body = the more fat you will burn according to John Rowley, Wellness Director for the International Sports Science Association.

You can imagine how fast you will lose fat combining Intermittent Fasting with a Keto diet and exercise plan

- **You are losing fat fast** without exercise and diet when you fast for 14-to-20 hours per day plus…

- **You are losing fat fast** when you eat less on your weight reduction diet.

- **You are losing fat fast** when you exercise *and if you exercise while you are fasting.*

You are going to burn fat much faster because your glucose levels are lower forcing your body to burn a lot more fat for energy as you workout.

2. **Intermittent Fasting increases your metabolism because as your glucose or energy levels get lower as you fast**.

- Your body reacts to this by re-energizing you by releasing more adrenaline which will make you to have more energy, be more alert and more focused but more importantly...

- As your body releases adrenaline it forces your body to burn fat **(mainly the stubborn fat on your thighs, belly and hips)** in order for you to get that much needed energy after your glucose drops and the theory to why your body does this is because.....

- Our ancestors (*like the Geico caveman*) would normally go through long unexpected fasting periods where their bodies would release adrenalin to give them the energy they needed to go hunting for the food they needed to survive.

3. Intermittent Fasting targets belly fat

Obstinate belly fat is difficult to lose simply because your abdominal region contains a lot more alpha-2 receptors **that hinder fat burning** than beta-2 receptors ***that speed up fat burning*** and because Intermittent Fasting reduces insulin...

- **Intermittent Fasting shuts off those a2 receptors** which do not work so well without insulin while activating more of the fat burning b2 receptors in your abdominal region permitting you to burn more stubborn belly fat.

Intermittent Fasting additionally increases blood flow to your abdominal region making it easier for your fat burning hormones (like adrenaline) to get into your abdominal region to **burn significantly more belly fat than normal diets.**

- With Intermittent Fasting **spot reduction is a reality** and not a myth more especially when you are trying to lose your last 10 pounds of stubborn fat.

Intermittent Fasting is more important for Women since women have much more stubborn fat or considerably more a2 receptors also in their hips, butt and thighs.

4. Intermittent Fasting naturally expands HGH (Human Growth Hormone)

HGH is a wonder hormone that burns fat, builds & maintains muscle mass.

Intermittent Fasting expands HGH by 2000% in Men and 1300% in women.

HGH keeps up your muscle mass while fasting and studies demonstrates that Intermittent Fasting diet does a better job (because of the extra HGH) of maintaining muscle mass versus other diets.

- There is no need to worry about losing any muscle mass while fasting

5. Intermittent Fasting makes you eat fewer calories

The less calories you eat = the faster you will lose weight.

When you first begin intermittent fasting the cravings and hunger will still be there but as YOU and YOUR body get acclimated to fasting... Your craving levels will go down and your cravings will eventually disappear because Intermittent fasting decreases or normalizes ghrelin (the hunger hormone) giving you less of an appetite.

With Intermittent Fasting you will most likely eat 1-to-3 meals daily depending upon how long your feasting period is and **you will actually Increase your hunger and cravings By NOT Intermittent Fasting** when you eat 3-to-6 meals a day as found in several studies.

Intermittent Fasting absolutely causes you to lose weight faster simply because...

- You are eating fewer calories due to less hunger and cravings.

- You are burning more fat/calories due to less insulin, more HGH and more adrenaline.

6 Tips on Intermittent Fasting

1. How to start intermittent fasting

Start bit by bit by fasting 12 hours per day or you can simply skip breakfast before working your way up to 14-to-20 hour day by day fast by adding an extra 15-to-30 minutes every day to your day by day fast.

- Once you are in the 16-to-20 plus hour range you will be in that perfect sweet spot for burning fat faster.

2. Best way to schedule your daily fast

When you are intermittent fasting you can plan your 14-to-20 hour fasting and 4-to-10 hour feasting cycle anyway you want to but for the best results **Its best that you eat your last meal 2-to-3 hours before bedtime** so you will spend less hours awake while you fast.

Most ideal approach to plan your every day fasting.

Here is an example of intermittent fasting schedule over a 24 hour time frame where you fast for 16 hours and eat over an 8 hour period...

Sunday night by 8pm: You stop eating your last meal.

- **Sunday night by 11pm**: You go to sleep (*so far you fasted for 3 hours*)

- **Monday morning by 7am**: You wake up (*so far you fasted for 11 hours*)

- **Monday between 7am-to-12pm:** You only spend 5 hours awake fasting

- **Monday by 12pm (noon): You have fasted a full 16 hours**

Monday from 12pm-to-8pm: You eat one or more meals at anytime during this period eating an exact amount of calories as lay out by your present diet plan.

Monday night at 8pm: You begin 16 hour fast

3. Eat whenever you want during your 4-to-10 hour feasting period

Most diets tell you **What to eat**, **When to eat**, and **How much to eat** and when you combine intermittent fasting with your current diet to burn fat faster...

The main change you will have to make is when you eat so you can still adhere to your diet plan but you need to eat all that you are supposed to within that 4-to-10 hour time frame and generally...

On a weight reduction diet you will eat under 1200-to-2000 calories everyday so you can get away with a shorter 4 hour feasting period with 1-to-2 meals.

- On muscle mass gaining diets you may eat more than 2000 calories per day so it is probably better for you to have a longer 8 hour feasting period with more than 2 meals to get all the carbs, protein and fats needed to build muscle

4. Managing hunger and cravings

It is going to take some time (possibly up to two days or a couple of weeks) until YOU and YOUR body becomes accustomed to Intermittent fasting and that is why it is best you start off just fasting 12 hours of the day by skipping breakfast.

If the hunger and cravings gets too intense and even headaches or dizziness occurs then break-your-fast, eat something, do not feel awful and simply try to fast a little longer until you hit the 16-to-20 hour range.

- **Tip:** Water or ZERO calorie coffee or green tea will help kill hunger and cravings while fasting.

5. Drink water, coffee and green tea

Intermittent fasting works simply because it FORCES your body to burn more fat by bringing down your blood sugar/ insulin levels by NOT EATING anything for 14-to-20 hours so...

- Drink all the water you need all through your 14-to-20 hour fasting period (*to help curb hunger*) since it contains ZERO calories.

- **Tip:** Drink ice cold water to lose weight faster.

- Coffee and green tea are okay during your fasting period as long as it is ZERO or very low calorie but you should really eat NO calories at all during your 14-to-20 hour fast to burn as much fat as possible *but on the other hand...*

- The caffeine in coffee and green tea accelerates your fat burning metabolism, it also forces your body to burn more fat and it curbs your appetite so that will offset the minor amount of calories you may get from coffee and green tea.

6. Workout while fasting

When your blood sugar, stored carbs/glycogen and insulin levels are lower from fasting **you will effortlessly burn more *fat* for energy** (*without any extra exercise or dieting*) so guess what happens when you exercise while you are fasting...

- You are going to burn a lot more fat when you workout and EVEN more fat when you do high intensity interval workouts (or HIIT) during your fasting time.

- **Tip:** Take a fat burner, ZERO-to-low calorie caffeinated coffee or green tea 30-to-60 minutes earlier than you begin your fasted workout to get an extra energy plus fat burning boost on top of the faster fat burning you are already getting from intermittent fasting.

- **If working out fasted scares you** Then simply schedule your workouts after you have had a meal during your 4-to-10 hour feasting period.

Why do we Accumulates more Fats These Days?

We live in a World where individuals use food for treatment rather than fuel. They eat when they are sad; People eat whenever they are happy. They eat when they are hungry and they even eat when they are full.

Eating is a nonstop activity and no thought is given as to what goes into their mouths.

As a result of this, their glucose levels are continuously spiking all through the day and the excess insulin that is secreted by the pancreas to adapt with the blood sugar levels gets converted to fat.

This is the main reason obesity has reached epidemic extents, and diabetes statistics have skyrocketed.

Intermittent fasting comprises of 2 windows: the fasting window and the eating window. During the eating window, which can be somewhere in the range of 5 to 8 hours, you will consume all your calories for the day.

During the fasting window, you will not consume any food at all. You may drink water, though. That is as simple as it gets... and this is what is called intermittent fasting in a nutshell. You are not starving, because you are still getting all the calories you need. This is a common misconception.

It seems difficult not to eat for 16 hours or so, but what most people do not realize is that you are fasting while you are asleep. All you need to do to fully experience the fast is by simply extend your fasting for a few more hours. A lot of people that have fasted intermittently have skipped only breakfast, and some have skipped dinner. Disregard the old adage about breakfast being the most important meal of the day.

Skipping breakfast and fasting for an additional 4 hours is actually quite beneficial and will assist you to lose excess fat.

You are not allowed to consume any food during your fast. Nevertheless, you can drink water and unsweetened green tea. Ideally, it is best to simply stick to water.

Why Do Millions Of People Do Intermittent Fasting?

Fasting has been around for so many years, and there is no indicated of it slowing down. There were times when people were forced to fast because food was scarce (during war times and economic recession).

Other than that, fasting is a practice in many different religions.

The Muslims fast during Ramadan, which allows the body to cleanse itself.

The Hindus fast before holy events for example Thaipoosam. If you read the

Bible, you had seen that Jesus fasted for 40 days and 40 nights too! Fasting is used as a way to develop discipline and as an approach to cleanse the body and achieve some degree of 'purity'.

Your body can withstand long periods of fasting and one of the major benefits of intermittent fasting are the cellular repair processes that your body experience.

During the fasting procedure, your glucose levels are decreased as well as your insulin level which makes it a perfect match to go alongside the Keto diet.

Your body can shed fat most effectively when there is very little glucose in the blood. Intermittent fasting assists you accomplish this state, and it is one of the main reasons your fat loss progress is accelerated.

Different Types of Fasting

Majority of people are not accustomed to go without food for a period of 16hrs. Let us not even talk about the more severe fasting diet that last from 24 to 48 hours.

To cure this little obstacle, there are numerous types of 'simpler' fasting procedure that they can adopt to see which suits them best.

As they build up the 'fasting muscle' they will be able to progress to the more advanced styles of fasting.

In this book, we will take a look at six popular fasting methods that are effective for weight reduction: **16/8 fast**

This is the most popular option for Individuals who have never practice fasting before and want to take it gradually.

You will be fasting for 16 hours and afterward eat within your allotted 8 hours (eating window). All you will be doing here is skipping one meal.

Most people prefer to skip breakfast, but this rule is not set in stone. If you MUST have breakfast to start your day, you may eat it. Just know that if you have breakfast at 8 am, your last meal of the day will have to be consumed by 4pm. This will ensure that you are fasting for 16 hours (from 4pm till 8am the following day).

For an Individual who works a 9 to 5 job, he/she will regularly skip breakfast, eat lunch at 12 noon and finish his/her last meal just before 8pm.

Fasting Within a Daily Window

There are numerous people who do not work from 9 to 5, and the fixed 16/8 style above is definitely not a good match for their schedule. If you are one of them, do not panic. Intermittent fasting can be adaptable.

The timings are NOT unchangeable. As long as your fasting duration is retained, the times of fasting can change.

Let us assume you have your breakfast at 10am and your last meal is just before 7pm – that means if you have breakfast at 10 am the following day, you had only fasted for 15hrs.

But what you are aiming for is a 16-hour fast, to comply with the 16/8 fast. In this case, all you will need to do is to extend the fast by another hour and just have your first meal at 11am. Now you had fasted for 16 hours. Your last meal can be at 7pm.

Keep doing this until you get to an 18-hour fasting window and this will give you the building blocks to try other fasting options.

Alternate Fasting

This is an amazingly strait forward protocol that is not really simple. All you will be doing is eating on one day and fasting the following day. It will look something like this: -

Monday: Fast

Tuesday: Eat

Wednesday: Fast

Thursday: Eat

Friday: Fast

Saturday: Eat

Sunday: Fast

Fasting for a full 24 hours can be a daunting task for some people and is best approached step by step. Aim for a few 18-hour fasts.

Gradually work your way up to 20-hour fasts.

When you are accustomed to fasting, you may attempt to go an entire 24 hours full fast. With this protocol you have two options:

• Do not eat anything except water. Not flavored water or water from the store but good old fashioned tap water.

(RECOMMENDED)

• If you are still new then this might be more appropriate for you. Maintain a caloric intake of around 500 – 600 calories on your fasting days also avoid sugar and starchy foods.

If this is the first time you want to do a 24-hour fast, aim for just two days out of every week in your first month. As you improve at it, you can go for more days or longer stretches.

Fat Fasting

If you are either looking to get started in the Keto diet or have fallen out of ketosis then this is the perfect option for you. Even if you have not seen any weight reduction since you began your

Keto diet, this method can certainly help to get your body back on track.

To get started, you will need to follow this procedure:

Eat only 1200 calories daily (for 3 days). Around 80-90% of calories in your diet should be made of fat. Divide your meals up into smaller portions and eat them all through the day (within your eating window). Some people adhere to bacon only for those three days while others take avocado and other foods that have good fat. After these 3 days, you will need to follow the rest of the keto diet rules while maintaining the intermittent fasting

procedure.

The Warrior Diet

This was founded by an ex-military expert called Ori Hofmekler, who eats as if he is an ancient warrior…live on one meal a day, which in those days was the hunt of the day.

There is no rigid dieting process to follow here apart from just going with your gut instinct and staying far away from processed foods.

Your fasting window is the entire day until night time where you can eat one large healthy meal. That basically means that you will be on an empty stomach throughout the whole day (water drinking is allowed) and just have one dinner daily.

24-Hour Fast

The name expresses it all. You fast for 24 hours and all you are allowed to consume is only water. That is it.

The time frame at which you begin is completely up to you. You can have lunch on Wednesday and afterward nothing until lunch time on Thursday.

You must remember always that: zero calories consumed during fasting. No coffee. No sugar free drinks. No energy drinks. ONLY WATER is permitted.

This style of fasting will get you into ketosis quickly and is highly effective for weight reduction. It requires discipline and battling the hunger pangs which come and go. However, if you can do it, you will be amazed at how much weight you will lose quickly.

Start off with the easier fasting procedures and work your way up to the 24-hour fasts.

Benefits of Intermittent Fasting

The major benefit of intermittent fasting that everyone talks widely about is the fast weight reduction. However, that is not the only benefit.

Actually, intermittent fasting does miracles for the body and there are many other benefits that can be gained from it. Let us look at what they are.

Ketosis

A very fast way to get your body to burn fat is to get it into a metabolic state called ketosis. When you are intermittent fasting, the body starts flushing out the glucose, and this will cause your insulin levels to fall drastically.

Once your insulin levels are very low, your body will then start to create ketones which will be your main source of energy. It will be easier to burn fat and you will feel more energetic too.

Autophagy

The cells in your body depreciate over time. This is actual duty of the ageing process. The deed of fasting actually sets your body in a state that is known as autophagy. When this happens, the body cleanses itself of worn out cells. The only thing that stops autophagy process is eating. When you eat, your body breaks the foods down into glucose which builds up insulin levels and stop the autophagy process.

Rejuvenates Skin

The most ideal approach to treat issues such as acne is by going on a clean diet and fasting intermittently for some weeks.

Eating just healthy foods during your eating window will leave you with radiant skin and you will look amazing. Not only that, intermittent fasting makes your hair and nails strong as well.

Brain Health

As you age, the brain gets less blood which brings about shrinking neurons and the volume of your brain declines. Intermittent fasting gives your brain a huge health boost and lowers down your risk of Parkinson's and Alzheimer's disease. Alzheimer's is additionally caused by obesity and intermittent fasting helps you to reduce your weight and diminish this potential cause.

Boosts Your Metabolism

Intermittent fasting will elevate your metabolism and help you burn more calories. As a result, not only will you be consuming fewer calories, but you will also be burning more fat.

Definitely a win win situation !!!

Longevity

Intermittent fasting enables you to live longer by shielding you from cancer and heart disease. It assists lower bad cholesterol levels, decreases insulin resistance and stabilizes your blood pressure.

If you currently have cancer and you are going through chemotherapy, intermittent fasting can help to build up your immune system.

Steps by Steps Instructions to Start Intermittent Fasting

You have made a wise choice to look after your health, and now it is time to get started.

1. Schedule your fast

Pick any day of the week to fast. Consider your present commitments like children, work and other must have activities before you decide on fasting.

2. Prepare your first fast

It is suggested that you speak to your doctor first to make sure that you do not have any complications that may disturb your health once you begin your fast.

En sure you understand why you are fasting. Is it for weight reduction, a detox or a short term thing?

3. Ease into fasting

There are various fasting procedures that you can adopt when you want to begin your fasting; however if this is your first time fasting, it is suggested that you begin with the 16/8 fast.

Different types of fasting methods mentioned in the previous chapters can be adopted when you have gained more experience.

In the event that you work a 2pm – 10pm shift, start your eating window during that time as you are on the move. Fast between 10pm and 2pm the next day. Work with your schedule and routine.

Things to Expect When Fasting

During the initial two days of your fasting, you will begin to feel exceptionally hungry. Most first timers to fasting will find out that they have less energy and are inclined to feeling moody and irritable.

Simply caution everybody around you to anticipate a grouchy you for the first two days! For the rest of the week, you will begin to notice a great changes in yourself and even physical changes in your body that will be noticeable by everybody. Depending on what your diet is, you may begin to enter ketosis during which your body becomes a fat-burning machine.

By the second week and going into the third week, you will see noticeable changes such as having a clearer mind, a good mood and having more energy. Your body is undergoing a healing process, and your immune system is being strengthened. You are being purified from the inside out.

By the fourth week, you will look and feel like a brand new you. Mental clearness, weight reduction, heightened senses and a better mood are general benefits of fasting. You will be amazed by how you look and feel. If you have taken the right steps all along, you ought to have accomplished your goals and are now on the path to living a healthy lifestyle.

How to Correctly End a Fast?

If you have been on a fast for a prolonged period, you need to deal with how you introduce more food into your body system. For every week you have been fasting you want to allow a period of two days to end your fast.

This normally takes time as your digestive system has gone through two things during a prolonged fast.

• Your stomach has contracted so much that eating even a smaller quantity of food can make you feel full.

• Your body has gotten a break from breaking down all the foods you used to eat during your fast, and it needs to be slowly woken up kind of like a grizzly bear.

You would prefer to wake them during winter. Wow! So, when you do end your fast, make sure you do it gradually and ease into it lightly.

If you have been fasting anywhere from 72 hours to 7 days, you will need to drink diluted foods and increase the quantities slowly over the first few days. Introduce fruit and milk in small quantities so as not to disturb your stomach.

As you gradually progress to solid foods, ensure you chew food slowly and to the point that it cannot be chewed anymore.

Rest and do not become active too soon. If you are working out, just stick to strolling. Do not engage in hard training. Give yourself sometime to recover.

When to Avoid Intermittent Fasting?
Intermittent fasting is an extraordinary method to lose weight. However, nothing is ideal for everybody; most importantly four groups of people below should avoid intermittent fasting.

• If you are underweight – If your BMI is below 18, at that point you do not have any extra body fat to burn off. There are numerous tutorials on how to calculate your BMI on Google.

• If you are pregnant – Your child is growing inside of you. So, do not restrict yourself from eating. You and your child need the nutrients. Eat healthy throughout and stay hydrated always.

• If you are breastfeeding – This would be the similar explanation as above except you would have given birth by now. Your body needs nutrients to produce milk to allow your baby to grow. Eat clean, eat well, and stay hydrated.

• If you are under 18 – Think once more…you are still growing. You will need all the right nutrients to reach your full potential. Eat well, be active and only fast if your religion requires it. Don't engage in intermittent Fasting.

Conclusion: Intermittent Fasting and Keto Diet

Without an iota of doubt, the keto diet and intermittent fasting are the perfect combinations when you want to lose weight and be in good shape.

You may find out about Individuals who have experienced some of the fantastic benefits that were covered. However, when you combined intermittent fasting with the keto diet and your results will skyrocket.

You will truly be taking things to the next level.

Give intermittent fasting a try. Once you have mastered it, you may adopt the keto diet and combine the two to burn up the remaining stubborn fat in your body.

You will then go from being overweight to having the body you have always dreamed of if you will make fasting and keto a part of your life style.

Get started today!